Praise for *The G.I. Diet* by Rick Gallop

"Losing weight is relatively easy with many 'fad' diets; maintaining the loss with these diets is difficult and largely impossible to sustain. Rick Gallop has found the key to permanent weight loss."

—Edmund H. Sonnenblick, M.D.
The Edmond J. Safra Professor of Medicine
and former Chief of Cardiology at the
Albert Einstein College of Medicine, New York City

"This diet is definitely the one that can help readers not only control weight but also help prevent cancer and heart disease."

—Elisabetta Politi, M.P.H., R.D., C.D.E., nutrition manager,
Duke University Diet and Fitness Center

"An innovative, realistic, uncomplicated, long-term approach to successful weight management."

—Michael Sole, M.D.,
Fellow of the American College of Cardiology

"Rick Gallop has been my diet coach for years, and now it's all here in a book that's easy, intelligent, and comes with exercises and nifty removable colored charts. This is my diet book forever."

—Barbara Amiel Black, columnist for
Chicago Sun-Times and *London Daily Telegraph*

"Dieting has never been made easier and more satisfying."

—Lucy Waverman, author and food columnist, *Globe & Mail*

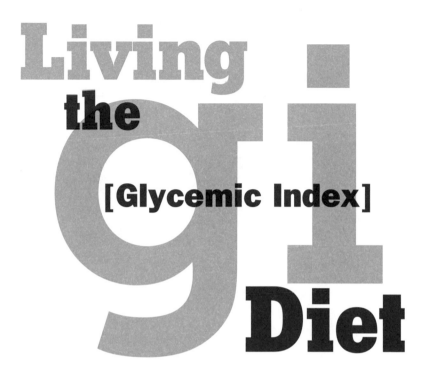

Living the gi [Glycemic Index] Diet

Delicious Recipes and Real-Life Strategies
TO LOSE WEIGHT AND KEEP IT OFF

RICK GALLOP

workman publishing • new york

First published in somewhat different form by
Random House Canada. This U.S. edition published
by arrangement with Random House Canada,
a division of Random House of Canada Limited.

Library of Congress Cataloging-in-Publication Data
is available.

ISBN 0-7611-3594-4

Design by Barbara Balch
Cover design by Paul Gamarello

Workman Publishing Company, Inc.
708 Broadway
New York, NY 10003-9555
www.workman.com

Printed in the United States of America

First printing December 2004

10 9 8 7 6 5 4 3 2 1

For the thousands of readers who have
shared their stories and success with me
and who gave me the inspiration and
motivation to write this book.

Contents

Introduction

In 2002 I published my first book, *The G.I. Diet*, with some trepidation. It wasn't the diet's effectiveness that I was worried about—far from it. I knew from personal experience that it was the best weight-loss program available. The book was based on the latest scientific research and had been endorsed by a number of physicians. I myself had even lost twenty pounds on it after nearly giving up hope of ever slimming down. What did concern me was that it might get lost in the sea of diet books crowding bookstore shelves—books that were full of empty promises, that promoted diets that were dangerously unhealthy, or that simply did not work.

I wanted to let people know the real cause of their weight problem and to show that they could lose the extra pounds easily, without having to perform difficult mathematical calculations or go hungry. I'm convinced that the reason Americans are gaining more weight than ever before is because they have simply been given the wrong information. The truth is you can eat as much as or even more than you currently do and still slim down. All you have to do is choose the right foods.

Fortunately, people took notice of *The G.I. Diet* and it clearly struck a chord with them. The book became a national bestseller in Canada, the United Kingdom, and the United States, and tens of thousands of readers have lost weight on the program! It is so rewarding to receive everyone's e-mails describing their successes—and they are the real motivation behind my writing this second book, *Living the G.I. Diet*. The biggest request by far was for more recipes, and that is exactly what this book contains—more than 140 delicious new recipes for breakfast, lunch, dinner, and between-meal snacks. Some are for everyday family dining, some are for entertaining, and some are for when time is short. I also wanted to provide even more information, with updated food lists, practical tips, FAQ's, and readers' letters along with these wonderful recipes to help you continue losing pounds or to maintain your new weight.

For those of you who didn't read *The G.I. Diet*, I've started this book with a short outline of its principles. This summary will give you everything you need to get started on the program right away. If you feel, however, that you need a more detailed explanation, you may want to read my first book. Those of you who are already familiar with the program can read the summary for a quick refresher or just skip over it. I should mention, though, that the G.I. Diet Food Guide on page 13 has been expanded to include more foods than appeared in the first book.

To further motivate you, I've shared some excerpts from the letters and e-mails I've received from people who are on the G.I. Diet. Their stories are often moving and truly inspiring. I am so proud of them and so grateful for their feedback. I hope that their experiences will help you as you embark on your journey to a new, slim you!

Please visit my Web site at **www.gidiet.com**
for the latest developments in nutrition and health.

Part One

The G.I. Diet Essentials

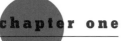

chapter one

The Secret to Easy, Permanent Weight Loss

For years doctors, nutritionists, and government groups have told us that the way to maintain a healthy weight is to eat a low-fat, high-carbohydrate diet. So if you've ever tried to lose weight, you've probably started by reducing the amount of fat that you eat. Instead of having bacon and eggs for breakfast, you switched to cornflakes with skim milk. Instead of eating a burger at lunch, you opted for a stuffed baked potato or a plain bagel without butter. Instead of snacking on potato chips, you munched on rice cakes. You made these healthier choices, felt good about yourself, and at the end of the month, you eagerly weighed yourself—to find that you'd gained another two pounds! What happened?

Well, first of all, let's dispel a widely held myth: Fat does not necessarily make you fat. Fat consumption in the United States has remained virtually constant over the past ten years, while obesity numbers have rocketed. Obviously fat isn't the real culprit. But that doesn't mean you can eat all the fatty foods you want. Most fats can be quite harmful to your health. It's alarming to read some of the popular diet books on the market today and find that they advocate eating lots of cream, cheese, and steak. These foods are all high in saturated fat, which can thicken arteries, leading to heart attack and stroke. There is also increasing evidence that colon and prostate cancer as well as Alzheimer's disease are associated with high levels of saturated fats. These are definitely the "bad" fats and are easily recognizable because they solidify at room temperature and almost always come from animal sources: butter, cheese, and high-fat meats like bacon and processed deli meats. There are two exceptions to this rule: Coconut oil and palm oil are two vegetable oils that are also saturated. Because these oils are cheap, they are used in many snack foods, especially cookies.

There is another, even worse fat category that I call the "really ugly" fats. The "really ugly" fats are potentially the most dangerous. They are vegetable oils that have been heat-treated to make them thicken. These hydrogenated oils or trans fatty acids take on the worst characteristics of saturated fats. So don't use them; and avoid foods whose labels list hydrogenated oils or partially hydrogenated oils among their ingredients. Many crackers, cereals, baked goods, and fast foods are the worst offenders, but U.S. food manufacturers won't be required to list the actual amounts of trans fatty acids in foods until 2006.

Avoiding the "bad" fats and the "really ugly" fats doesn't mean eliminating fat entirely from our diet. Fortunately, there are a number of healthy fat options, too. Fats are absolutely essential to our health because they contain various key elements that are crucial to the digestive process. The "best" fats are monounsaturated fats, which are found in foods like olives, peanuts, almonds, and olive and canola oils. Monounsaturated fats actually have a beneficial effect on cholesterol and are good for your heart. So try to incorporate them into your diet and look for them on food labels. Most manufacturers who use them will say so, because they know it's a key selling point for informed consumers.

Another highly beneficial oil, which is in a category of its own, contains a wonderful ingredient called omega-3. This oil is found in coldwater fish such as salmon, and in flax seeds and canola oil, and it's extremely good for your heart health. "Acceptable" fats are the polyunsaturated fats because they are cholesterol free. Most vegetable oils, such as corn, safflower, and sunflower, fall into this category.

So what exactly causes people to gain weight if it isn't fat? Well, the answer lies in something you've probably never thought of as fattening at all—and that's grain. Have you noticed the multiplying number of grocery store shelves dedicated to products made from flour, corn, and rice? Supermarkets now have huge cracker, cookie, and snack food sections; whole aisles of cereals; numerous shelves of pastas and noodles; and baskets and baskets of bagels, rolls, muffins, and loaves of bread. In 1970 the average North American ate about 135 pounds of grain. By 2000 that figure had risen to nearly *200* pounds! This staggering increase helps explain why 61 percent of American adults are overweight, and why one in four are considered obese—that's double the amount twenty years ago! We're definitely eating too much grain, but the other half of the problem is the *type* of grain we're eating, which is generally highly processed. Take flour, for instance. Today's high-speed flour mills use steel rollers rather than traditional grinding stones to produce an extraordinarily finely ground product. The whole wheat is steamed and scarified by tiny razor-sharp blades to remove the bran and the endosperm. Then the wheat germ and oil are removed because they turn rancid too quickly to last on supermarket shelves. What's left after all that processing is then bleached and marketed as all-purpose flour. This is what almost all the breads, bagels, muffins, cookies, crackers, cereals, and pastas we consume are made of. Even many "brown" breads are simply artificially colored white bread.

And it's not just flour that's highly processed nowadays. A hundred years ago most of the food people ate came straight from the farm to the dinner table. Lack of refrigeration and scant knowledge of food chemistry meant that most food remained in its original state. However, advances in science, along with the migration

GRAIN CONSUMPTION (POUNDS PER CAPITA)

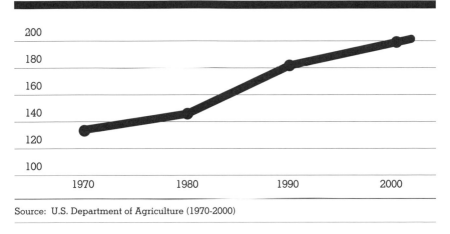

Source: U.S. Department of Agriculture (1970-2000)

of many women out of the kitchen and into the workforce, led to a revolution in prepared foods. Everything became geared to speed and simplicity of preparation. We now have instant rice and potatoes, as well as entire meals that are ready to eat after just a few minutes in the microwave.

The trouble with all this is that the more a food is processed beyond its natural state, the less processing your body has to do to digest it. And the quicker you digest your food, the sooner you are hungry again and the more you tend to eat. The difference between eating a bowl of old-fashioned, slow-cooking oatmeal and a bowl of sugary cold cereal is that the oatmeal stays with you—it "sticks to your ribs" as my mother used to say—whereas you are looking for your next meal only an hour after eating the bowl of sugary cereal. Our fundamental problem, then, is that we are eating foods that are digested by our bodies too easily. Clearly we can't wind back the clock to simpler times, but we need to somehow slow down the digestive process so we feel hungry less often. How can we do that? Well, we have to eat foods that are *slow-release*, that break down at a *slow and steady rate* in our digestive system, leaving us feeling fuller for longer.

There are two clues to identifying slow-release foods. The first is the amount of fiber in the food. Fiber, in simple terms, provides low-calorie filler. It does double duty, in fact, by literally filling up your stomach so that you feel satiated, and by taking much longer to break down in your body, so the digestive process is slowed and the food stays with you longer. There are two forms of fiber: soluble and insoluble. Soluble fiber is found in foods like oatmeal, beans, barley, and citrus fruits, and has been shown to lower blood cholesterol levels. Insoluble fiber is important for normal bowel function and is typically found in whole wheat breads and cereals and most vegetables.

The second tool in identifying slow-release foods is the glycemic index, or G.I. The G.I. is the secret to successful weight management and the basis of the G.I. Diet, which I developed in 2002. The glycemic index itself is the result of research undertaken by Dr. David Jenkins, a professor of nutrition at the University of Toronto. Early in his career, Dr. Jenkins became interested in diabetes, a disease that hampers the body's ability to process carbohydrates and sugar (glucose). Sugar therefore stays in the bloodstream instead of going into the body's cells, resulting in hyperglycemia and potentially coma. At the time Dr. Jenkins was beginning his research, carbohydrates were severely restricted in a diabetic's diet because they quickly boost the sugar level in the bloodstream. But because the primary role of carbohydrates is to provide the body with energy, diabetics were having to make up the lack of calories through a high-fat diet, which provides energy without boosting sugar levels. Now doctors were in a real quandary; although they were saving diabetics from hyperglycemia, they were accelerating their risk of heart disease.

Dr. Jenkins wondered if all carbohydrates are the same. Are some digested more quickly, and do they therby raise blood sugar levels faster than others? And are others slow-release, resulting in only a marginal incrcasc in blood sugar? The answer to both questions, he discovered, is yes. In 1980, he published an index—the glycemic index—showing the various rates at which carbohydrates break down and release glucose into the bloodstream. The faster the food breaks down, the higher the rating on the index, which sets pure glucose (sugar) at 100 and scores all other foods against that number. The chart on the next page contains some examples of G.I. ratings.

By eating only those foods that have a low G.I. rating, diabetics were now able to reintroduce a number of carbohydrates to their diets while keeping their glucose levels low and avoiding hyperglycemia.

THE PERMANENT WEIGHT-LOSS SOLUTION

As it turns out, the G.I. also has exciting implications for anyone who wishes to lose weight. It has been proven that keeping glucose levels low is the key to permanent weight loss. This is how it works: When you eat a high-G.I. food, your body rapidly converts it into glucose. The glucose dissolves in your bloodstream and spikes its glucose level, giving you that "sugar high."

After your glucose level spikes, it quickly disappears from your bloodstream, leaving you feeling starved of energy and looking for

"I started the G.I. Diet on April 1, at which point I weighed 150 pounds, and by September 1, I had reached my target of 134 pounds. I have nonsustained ventricular tachycardia, controlled by medication, and see my cardiologist each year for a checkup. She was impressed by my achievement and told me that this year, I was fitter than I had been on any of my previous visits and that my blood pressure, which has never been high, was reduced as a result."

—Stan

G.I. RATINGS OF SELECTED FOODS

glucose(sugar) = 100

Baguette	95	Orange	44
Rice (instant)	87	All-Bran	43
Cornflakes	84	Oatmeal	42
Potatoes (baked)	84	Peach	42
Doughnut	76	Spaghetti	41
Cheerios	75	Apple	38
Bagel	72	Tomato	38
Raisins	64	Yogurt (low-fat)	33
Rice (basmati)	58	Fettuccine	32
Muffin (bran)	56	Beans	31
Potatoes (new, boiled)	56	Grapefruit	25
Popcorn (microwave light)	55	Yogurt (nonfat with sweetener)	14

more fuel. Something most of us experience regularly is the feeling of lethargy that follows an hour or so after a fast-food lunch, which generally consists of high-G.I. foods. The surge of glucose followed by the rapid drain leaves us feeling sluggish and hungry. So what do we do? Around mid-afternoon we look for a quick sugar fix, or snack, to bring us out of the slump. A few cookies or a bag of chips—also high-G.I. foods—cause another rush of glucose, which again disappears a short time later. And so the vicious circle continues. Eating a diet of high-G.I. foods will obviously make you feel hungry more often and you will end up eating more as a result. Low-G.I. foods, on the other hand, are the tortoise to the high-G.I. foods' hare. They break down in your digestive system at a slow, steady rate. Tortoiselike, they stay the course, making you feel full longer, and consequently, you eat less. The chart on page 9 illustrates the impact of digesting sugar on the level of glucose in your bloodstream compared with Cheerios, another high-G.I. food, and oatmeal, which has a low G.I. rating.

There is a second reason why you should avoid eating high-G.I. foods when you are trying to lose weight. When you experience a rapid spike in your blood sugar, your pancreas releases the hormone insulin. Insulin does two things extremely well. First, it reduces the level of glucose in your bloodstream by diverting it into various body tissues for immediate short-term use or by storing it as fat—which is why glucose disappears so quickly. Second, it inhibits the conversion of body fat back into glucose for the body to burn. This evolutionary feature is a throwback to the days when our ancestors were hunter-gatherers, habitually experiencing times of feast or famine. When food was in abundance, the body stored its surplus as fat to tide it over the days when there wouldn't be much to eat. Insulin was the champion in this process, both helping to accumulate fat and then guarding its depletion.

Today, everything has changed but our stomachs. We don't have to hunt for food anymore—there's a guaranteed supply at the supermarket. But our insulin continues to store fat and keep it intact. Our bodies must be able to access and burn away our fat cells in order to lose weight. To allow that to happen, you need to do two things. First, you must consume fewer calories than your body needs in order to burn up those fat stores. Now, I hate to

G.I. IMPACT ON BLOOD SUGAR

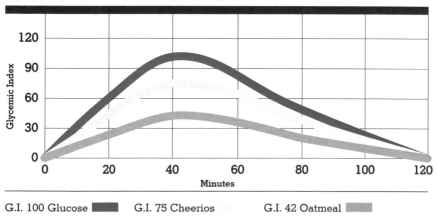

G.I. 100 Glucose ▇▇   G.I. 75 Cheerios   G.I. 42 Oatmeal ▒▒

bring up calories since we've probably all been driven nearly over the edge by having to count them and even perform complex mathematical calculations with them. But unfortunately, unless one denies the basic laws of thermodynamics, the equation never changes: Consume more calories than you expend, and the surplus is stored in the body as fat. That's the inescapable fact. Few diet books today mention calories, but they're there, hidden behind the various rules and suggestions. Don't worry, though, because with *Living the G.I. Diet* you can easily reduce your calorie intake without having to do any calculations and without going hungry. I'll explain how in a moment.

> *"Your diet rocks!! We're never hungry, we can't believe the gradual and constant weight loss, and we can't believe that we can eat out, travel, celebrate special events, and still, albeit sometimes partially, stick to the regime and keep the weight off. I've spent the last two days taking my husband's pants, shorts, and shirts in—some of them 4½ inches! He's a happy guy, and I'm the happy girl who can reach all the way around him and hug him to death."*
>
> *—Joann*

CHOOSING LOW-G.I. FOODS INSTEAD OF HIGH-G.I. FOODS

The second thing we must do to enable our bodies to use up their fat cells is to keep our insulin levels low, which means avoiding high-G.I. foods. Remember the cornflakes, baked potato, plain bagel, and rice cakes that were mentioned at the beginning of this chapter? Well, you would never lose weight if you ate those foods on a daily basis because they all have high G.I. ratings: They raise your insulin levels to the point where your body won't burn up those fat stores. Instead, you should stick to low-G.I. foods. Instead of having cornflakes for breakfast, have large-flake (old-fashioned) oatmeal or homemade muesli. Instead of lunching on a big bagel, enjoy a bowl of homemade lentil soup. Avoid the rice cakes when you need a snack, and have a handful of hazelnuts or almonds instead. It isn't difficult to substitute low-G.I. foods for high-G.I. ones, and by making these changes, you will begin to see your weight drop. It's that easy.

How will you know which foods are high-G.I. and which ones are low? In the next chapter you'll find a comprehensive chart that identifies the foods that will make you fat and those that will allow you to lose weight. Don't expect the foods in the latter category to be limited and boring; there are so many tasty and satisfying choices that you won't even feel as though you are on a diet. And later in this book I'll give you many delicious ways to prepare these foods.

"I absolutely love this plan and find it so easy to live with. My husband and I can still go out to eat and not feel like I am deprived of food or fun! I have started a lot of my coworkers (all in the medical field) on this plan, and they have also had success."
—Merrill

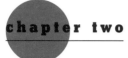

chapter two

The G.I. Diet

Now that you understand the principles behind the G.I. Diet, it's time to get down to the nitty-gritty. Basically, this chapter addresses what, when, and how much to eat to start shedding those extra pounds. Let's begin by addressing the "what." As you know from the last chapter, the key to losing weight is to eat foods that have two essential characteristics: a low calorie content and a low G.I. rating. To help you identify those foods, I have developed an easy-to-use reference tool called the G.I. Diet Food Guide.

THE G.I. DIET FOOD GUIDE

This chart lists every food you can think of in one of three categories based on the colors of a traffic light. Foods listed in the red-light or "stop" category are high-G.I., high-calorie foods that should be avoided. Some of these may surprise you—for example, melba toast, white rice, turnips, and watermelon are all red-light. They may be low in fat, but your body digests them so quickly that you are hungry again an hour later. Foods in the yellow-light or "caution" category—for example, sourdough bread, corn, and bananas—have moderate G.I. ratings, but they do raise insulin levels to the point where weight loss is not going to happen. Foods in the green-light or "go ahead" category are the ones that will allow you to lose weight. Chicken, long-grain rice, and asparagus are all green-light foods. Eat them and watch your weight drop. After you've had a chance to look over the G.I. Diet Food Guide, we'll talk about how to make it work for you.

THE COMPLETE G.I. DIET FOOD GUIDE

	● RED LIGHT	YELLOW LIGHT	● GREEN LIGHT
beans	Baked beans with pork Fava (broad) beans Refried beans	Kidney beans (canned) Lentils (canned)	Baked beans (low-fat)* Black beans Black-eyed peas Chickpeas Italian beans Kidney beans Lentils Lima/butter beans Mung beans Navy/haricot beans Peas Pigeon beans Pinto beans Soybeans Split peas
beverages	Alcoholic drinks (in general) Fruit juices (sweetened)	Beer** Coffee (with skim milk, no sugar) Diet soft drinks (caffeinated)	Bottled water Club soda Decaffeinated coffee (with skim milk, no sugar)

*Limit quantity.

**In Phase II, a glass of wine and an occasional beer may be included. Red wine in moderation has been shown to have cardiovascular benefits.

	● RED LIGHT	YELLOW LIGHT	● GREEN LIGHT
beverages (continued)	Regular soft drinks	Fruit juices (unsweetened) (see page 29) Light instant chocolate drinks Vegetable juice cocktails (e.g., V8) Wine (preferably red)*	Diet soft drinks (no caffeine) Herbal tea Tea (with skim milk, no sugar)
breads	Bagels Baguette/ croissants Cake/cookies Cornbread English muffins Hamburger buns Hot dog buns Kaiser rolls Melba toast Muffins/ doughnuts Pancakes/ waffles Pizza Regular granola bars Stuffing Tortillas White bread	Crisp breads with fiber Pita bread (whole wheat) Sourdough bread Tortillas (low-carb) Whole grain breads	Crisp breads with high fiber Homemade muffins (see pages 261–268) Homemade pancakes (see pages 100–105) 100% stone-ground whole-wheat bread** Whole-grain, high fiber bread**

*See Alcohol, page 55.

**Limit quantity (see page 24).

	RED LIGHT	YELLOW LIGHT	GREEN LIGHT
cereal grains	Millet Polenta Quinoa Rice (short-grain, white, instant) Rice cakes	Corn	Barley Buckwheat Bulgur Gram flour Rice (basmati, brown, long-grain, wild) Wheat berries
cereals	All cold cereals except those listed as yellow or green light Cream of Wheat Granola Grits Muesli (commercial) Instant/quick-cook oatmeal	Kashi Go Lean Crunch Kashi Good Friends Shredded Wheat Bran	All-Bran Bran Buds 100% Bran Fiber Fiber One Homemade Muesli (page 96) Kashi Go Lean Large-flake oatmeal (e.g., Quaker Old-Fashioned Oats) Oat bran
condiments/ seasonings	Croutons Ketchup Mayonnaise Tartar sauce	Mayonnaise (light)	Chili powder Extracts (vanilla, etc.) Garlic Herbs/spices Hummus Lemon/lime juice Mayonnaise (fat-free) Mustard

	RED LIGHT	YELLOW LIGHT	GREEN LIGHT
condiments/ seasonings (continued)			Salsa (low-sugar) Soy sauce (low-sodium) Teriyaki sauce Vinegar Worcestershire sauce
dairy	Almond milk Cheese Chocolate milk Cottage cheese (whole or 2%) Cream Cream cheese Evaporated milk Ice cream Milk (whole or 2%) Rice milk Sour cream Yogurt (whole or 2%)	Cheese (low-fat) Cream cheese (light) Frozen yogurt (low-fat, low-sugar) Ice cream (low-fat) Milk (1%) Sour cream (light) Yogurt (low-fat with sugar)	Buttermilk Cheese (fat-free or extra low-fat; e.g., Laughing Cow Light, Boursin Light) Cottage cheese (1% or fat-free) Cream cheese (nonfat) Ice cream* (low-fat and no added sugar) Milk (skim) Frozen yogurt (nonfat and no added sugar) Fruit yogurt (nonfat with sweetener) Sour cream (fat-free) Soy cheese (low-fat) Soy milk, plain (low-fat) Soy/whey protein powder

*Limit quantity (see page 307).

	● RED LIGHT	YELLOW LIGHT	● GREEN LIGHT
eggs	Regular eggs	Omega-3 eggs	Liquid eggs Egg Beaters Egg whites
fats/oils	Butter Coconut oil Hard margarine Lard Mayonnaise Palm oil Salad dressings (regular) Tropical oils Vegetable shortening	Corn oil Mayonnaise (light) Peanut oil Salad dressings (light) Sesame oil Soft margarine (nonhydro-genated) Soy oil Sunflower oil Vegetable oil	Canola oil*/seed Flax seed/flax oil Mayonnaise (fat-free) Olive oil* Salad dressings (low-fat, low-sugar) Soft margarine* (nonhydro-genated, light; e.g., Promise Ultra) Vegetable oil sprays Vinaigrette
fish/ shellfish	Breaded/battered Sushi rolls	Canned in oil	All fresh, canned, frozen Sashimi Smoked salmon
fruits (fresh)	Cantaloupe Dates Honeydew melon Melons Prunes Watermelon	Apricots Bananas Custard apples Fruit cocktail (in juice) Kiwis Mangoes	Apples Blackberries Blueberries Cherries Grapefruit Grapes Guavas

*Limit quantity (see page 24).

	● RED LIGHT	YELLOW LIGHT	● GREEN LIGHT
fruits (fresh) (continued)		Papayas Pineapple Pomegranates	Lemons Nectarines Oranges (all varieties) Peaches Pears Plums Raspberries Rhubarb Strawberries
fruits (bottled, canned, frozen, dried)	Applesauce containing sugar Most canned fruit in syrup Most dried fruit* Raisins* Regular fruit spread	Apricots Dried apricots* Dried cranberries* Fruit cocktail in juice	Applesauce (unsweetened) Extra-fruit, low-sugar spreads Frozen berries Mandarin oranges Peaches/pears in juice or water
fruit juices**	All fruit drinks All sweetened juices Prune Sorbet Watermelon	Apple (unsweetened) Cranberry (unsweetened) Grapefruit (unsweetened) Orange (unsweetened) Pear (unsweetened) Pineapple (unsweetened)	

*For baking, it is okay to use a modest amount of dried fruits.

**Whenever possible, eat the fruit rather than drink its juice.

	● RED LIGHT	YELLOW LIGHT	● GREEN LIGHT
meats: **beef**	Brisket Regular ground Short ribs	Lean ground (10%–20% fat) Sirloin Sirloin tips T-bone Tenderloin	Extra-lean ground (less than 10% fat) Eye round Top round
lamb	Rack	Fore shank Center cut Leg shank Loin chop	
pork **(fresh)**	Back ribs Blade Spare ribs	Center loin Fresh ham Shank Sirloin Top loin	Tenderloin
pork **(cured)**	Bacon strips		Canadian bacon Ham (extra-lean)
veal			Blade steak Cutlet Loin chop Rib roast Shank
processed **meats**	Bologna (all meats) Hot dogs Pastrami (beef) Salami Sausages	Corned beef Dried beef	Ham (deli-style) Pastrami (turkey) Turkey breast Turkey roll

	● RED LIGHT	YELLOW LIGHT	● GREEN LIGHT
other meats	Organ meats Offal Pâté		
nuts/seeds	Peanut butter (regular/light)	100% nut butters Peanuts Pecans 100% peanut butter Sunflower seeds Walnuts	Almonds* Cashews* Flax seed Hazelnuts* Macadamia nuts* Pistachios* Soy nuts*
pasta**	All canned pastas Couscous Gnocchi Macaroni and cheese Noodles (canned/instant) Pasta filled with cheese or meat	Rice noodles	Capellini Cellophane (mung bean) noodles Fettuccine Linguine Macaroni Penne Rigatoni Spaghetti Vermicelli
pasta sauces	Alfredo sauces with added meat or cheese Sauces with added sugar or sucrose	Sauces with vegetables	Light sauces with vegetables (no added sugar; e.g., Healthy Choice, Colavita, Classico)

*Limit quantity (see page 24).

**Use whole-wheat or protein-enriched pastas if available. Limit quantity (see page 24).

	● RED LIGHT	YELLOW LIGHT	● GREEN LIGHT
poultry: chicken/ turkey	Breast with skin Roasters/stewing light /dark with skin Thigh with skin Wing with skin	Roasters/stewing light /dark without skin Thigh without skin Turkey bacon	Breast without skin
other poultry	Duck (all parts) Goose (all parts)		
snacks	Bagels Bread Candy Cookies Crackers Doughnuts French fries Ice cream Instant pudding Jell-O Muffins (commercial) Popcorn (regular) Potato chips Pretzels Raisins Rice cakes Tortilla chips Trail mix	Bananas Dark chocolate* (70% cocoa) Ice cream (low-fat) Most nuts Popcorn (light, microwavable/ air-popped)	Applesauce (unsweetened) Canned peaches/ pears in juice or water Cottage cheese (1% or fat-free) Frozen yogurt (nonfat and no added sugar) Fruit Yogurt (nonfat with sweetener) Green-light nuts and seeds (see page 20) Homemade Muffins (see pages 261–268) Ice cream (low-fat and no added sugar)

*Limit quantity (see page 24).

	● RED LIGHT	YELLOW LIGHT	● GREEN LIGHT
snacks (continued)			Most fresh fruit (see page 17) Most fresh vegetables (see page 23) Soy nuts Sugar-free gum/candy
soups	All cream-based soups Canned black bean Canned green/split pea Pureed vegetable	Canned chicken noodle Canned lentil Canned tomato	All homemade soups made with green-light ingredients Chunky bean and vegetable canned soups (e.g., Campbell's Healthy Request and Healthy Choice)
soy meat substitutes		Tofu (regular)	Tofu (low-fat) TVP (textured vegetable protein) Veggie burger
sugar and sweeteners	Corn syrup Glucose Honey Molasses Sugar (all types)	Fructose	Aspartame Brown sugar substitute (e.g. Sugar Twin) Equal Splenda Stevia* Sugar Twin Sweet'n Low

*Note: Not FDA approved.

	● RED LIGHT	YELLOW LIGHT	● GREEN LIGHT
vegetables	French fries	Artichokes	Collard greens
	Hash browns	Beets	Cucumbers
	Parsnips	Corn	Eggplant
	Potatoes (instant/mashed/ baked)	Potatoes (boiled)	Kale
		Pumpkin	Kohlrabi
	Rutabagas	Squash	Leeks
	Turnips	Sweet potatoes	Lettuce (all varieties)
		Yams	Mushrooms
			Mustard greens
			Okra
		Alfalfa sprouts	Olives*
		Arugula	Onions
		Asparagus	Peas
		Avocado	Peppers (hot)
		Beans (green/wax)	Pickles
		Bell peppers	Potatoes (boiled new)*
		Bok choy	Radiccio
		Broccoli	Radishes
		Brussels sprouts	Sauerkraut
		Cabbage	Snow peas
		Capers	Spinach
		Carrots	Swiss chard
		Cauliflower	Tomatoes
		Celery	Zucchini

*Limit quantity (see page 24).

SERVINGS AND PORTIONS

The G.I. Diet Food Guide makes choosing the right foods for your new eating plan easy. But how much of them should you eat and when? First of all, this isn't a deprivation diet. For the most part, you can have as much of the green-light foods as you like. There are only a few exceptions, which have a higher G.I. rating or calorie content than others. I've listed them along with their recommended serving sizes below.

GREEN-LIGHT SERVINGS

Food	Recommended Serving Size
Green-light breads (at least 2½ to 3 grams of fiber per slice)	1 slice
Green-light cereals	½ cup
Green-light nuts	8 to 10
Margarine (nonhydrogenated, light)	2 teaspoons
Meat, fish, poultry	4 ounces (about the size of a deck of cards)
Olive or canola oil	1 teaspoon
Olives	4 or 5
Pasta	¾ cup cooked
Potatoes (boiled new)	2 to 3
Rice (basmati, brown, long-grain)	⅔ cup cooked
Phase II (weight maintenance)	
Chocolate (70% cocoa)	2 squares
Red wine	1 glass (5 ounces)

Some readers have asked me if it's okay to eat twelve apples a day or an entire tub of cottage cheese at a sitting! I don't recommend that you go overboard on quantities of anything. Moderation is key. It's also important that you spread your daily calorie intake evenly throughout the day. If your digestive system is busy processing food and steadily supplying energy to your brain, you won't be desperately looking for high-calorie snacks. I know that many people make a habit of skipping breakfast in the morning, but this is a big mistake. People who miss breakfast leave their stomachs empty from dinner to lunch the next day, often more than sixteen hours! No wonder they overeat at lunch and then look for a sugar fix at mid-afternoon as they run out of steam. Always eat three meals—breakfast, lunch, and dinner—as well as three snacks—one mid-morning, one mid-afternoon, and one before bed—each day. And try to consume approximately the same amount of calories at each principal meal. If you eat a tiny breakfast and then a tiny lunch, you'll feel so hungry by dinnertime that you won't be able to stop yourself from overeating.

As well, each meal should contain some vegetables or fruit, some protein, and some type of whole-grain food. Fruits, vegetables, and grains are all carbohydrates, which are the primary source of energy for your body. They are rich in fiber, vitamins, and minerals, including antioxidants, which we now believe play a critical role in protecting against disease—especially heart disease and cancer. That's one of the reasons why high-protein, low-carb diets, which unfortunately have become quite popular in recent years, are so harmful to your long-term health. They prescribe eating a

"At age 35, I was 320 pounds with a family history of diabetes. To make matters worse, I broke my ankle and spent last summer on the couch, and was diagnosed with severe sleep apnea. My wife and I have been on the G.I. Diet since January [five weeks], and if I continue losing at this rate I will be at my high school weight (185) and a normal BMI by August. I feel so empowered."
—Derek

USDA FOOD PYRAMID

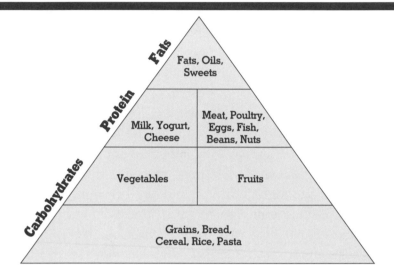

Source: U.S. Department of Agriculture

THE G.I. DIET FOOD PYRAMID

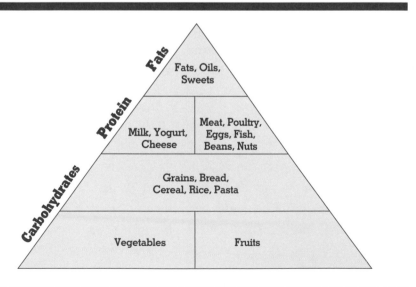

TRADITIONAL   G.I. DIET

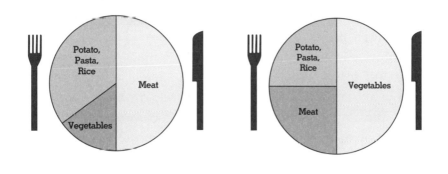

great deal of animal protein, which is high in saturated fat, while severely cutting back on carbohydrates. This causes ketosis, a dangerous electrolyte imbalance and an acid buildup in the blood that can lead to kidney damage, kidney stones, and osteoporosis. Side effects include fatigue, headache, nausea, dizziness, and bad breath. By minimizing the amount of vegetables, fruits, whole grains, and legumes you consume, you deprive your body of essential vitamins and minerals. So the issue we should be concerned about is not "low carbs" but rather selecting "good carbs," which are nutritious and will help you lose weight.

With that in mind, vegetables and fruits, most of which are low-calorie and low-G.I., form the base of the G.I. Diet. Now, I know that the current U.S. Department of Agriculture's Food Pyramid suggests that grains should be the largest component of your diet, followed by vegetables and fruit. But by giving grains priority, the USDA is promoting the leading cause of overweight and obesity. Recently, the Mayo Clinic, one of the world's leading medical research centers, has begun to promote vegetables and fruits, rather than grains, as the basis of a healthy diet.

Protein is another essential part of your diet. Half of your dry body weight is made up of protein, including your muscles, organs, skin, and hair, and protein is required to build and repair body tissue. It is also much more effective than carbohydrates or fat in satisfying hunger. It acts as a brake in the digestive process and will make you feel fuller longer, as well as more alert. So while I don't support high-protein, low-carb diets, you should definitely include some protein in every meal. Too often we grab a hasty breakfast of coffee and toast—a protein-free meal. Lunch is sometimes not much better: a bowl of pasta, a cup of soup, or a green salad and bread. And a typical afternoon snack of a cookie, a piece of fruit, or a bag of potato chips contains not a gram of protein. Generally, it's not until dinner that we eat protein, usually our entire daily recommended allowance plus some extra. But because protein is a critical brain food, providing amino acids for the neurotransmitters that relay messages in the brain, it would be better to load up on it earlier in the day. That would give you an alert and active mind for your daily activities.

The best solution, however, is to spread your protein consumption throughout the day to keep you on the ball and feeling full. Choose low-fat proteins such as lean or low-fat meats that have been trimmed of any visible fat; skinless poultry; fresh, frozen, or canned fish and shellfish (but not the kind that's coated in batter, which is invariably high in unhealthy fat); beans; low-fat dairy products like skim milk (believe it or not, after a couple of weeks of drinking it, it tastes just like 2%), low-fat yogurt without sugar, and low-fat cottage cheese; low-cholesterol liquid eggs; and tofu.

"When I have to eat other food that's not on the G.I. Diet, I am amazed at how quickly I need to sleep in the afternoon and how little energy I have. Now that is the exception rather than the rule. I can't understand why anybody even looks at any other diet when this is the only one that really works."
—Daphne

An easy way to visualize the portion sizes you should be consuming is to imagine your plate divided into three sections. Half the plate should be covered with vegetables and fruit. One of the sources of protein listed above should occupy one quarter of the plate, and the last quarter should be filled with a green-light type of rice, pasta, potato, or cooked whole grain. On page 27 is a diagram of what your green-light dinner plate should look like.

WHAT TO HAVE FOR BREAKFAST

To make your regular breakfasts green-light, here are some general guidelines to follow.

Coffee

The principal problem with coffee is its caffeine content. There is growing evidence to suggest that caffeine causes your body to produce high levels of insulin—which is the last thing we want. That's why I recommend you drink only decaffeinated coffee when you are trying to lose weight. If you simply can't face the day without a cup of java, caffeine intact, then please, go ahead and have it. But don't add sugar—use a sugar substitute instead—and add only 1% or skim milk. I have received so many e-mails from readers who feel that caffeine deprivation is a definite deal breaker. If you follow the other principles of the G.I. Diet, you can have your morning cup of coffee and still reach your weight-loss target.

Juice/Fruit

Always eat the fruit rather than drink its juice. Juice is a processed product that is more rapidly digested than the parent fruit. To illustrate the point, diabetics who run into an insulin crisis and are in a state of hypoglycemia (low blood sugar) are usually given orange juice because it's the fastest way to get glucose into the bloodstream. A glass of juice has two and a half times the calories of a fresh whole orange.

Oatmeal

My favorite breakfast of all time is good old-fashioned oatmeal. Not only is it low-G.I. and low-calorie, but it also lowers cholesterol. Be sure to use the large-flake variety, also called old-fashioned style, and not the one-minute or instant oats, which have been processed. Oatmeal will stay with you all morning and it is easy to prepare, especially in the microwave. You can also endlessly vary the flavor by adding nonfat, sugar-free, fruit-flavored yogurt; unsweetened applesauce; nuts; or fruit.

Cereals

Go for the high-fiber products that have at least 10 grams of fiber per serving. Oat bran is also excellent. Though these cereals are not much fun in and of themselves, you can liven them up with fresh or canned fruit, nuts, and nonfat, sugar-free, fruit-flavored yogurt. You can also add sweetener (though stay away from sugar).

Toast

Always use bread that has 2½ to 3 grams of fiber per slice. Many of the nutrient content labels on breads list fiber for a two-slice serving—remember, however, that a green-light serving is only *one slice* per meal, and evaluate labels accordingly. A good choice of bread is 100% stone-ground whole wheat. "Stone-ground" means the flour has been ground with stones rather than steel rollers, resulting in a coarser grind and a lower G.I. rating.

Spreads

Do not use butter. The premium brands of nonhydrogenated soft margarine are acceptable, and the light versions are even more so, but still use them sparingly. And look for the "extra-fruit/sugar-reduced" versions of fruit spreads. These taste terrific and are very low in calories. Regular jelly, jam, and preserves are just too sugar-packed. Avoid all brands in which the first ingredient listed is sugar.

Eggs

By far the best option is whole eggs in liquid form (such as Egg Beaters), which you can buy in cartons in the egg and dairy section of your grocery store. Because the fat and cholesterol levels have been reduced, liquid eggs are great green-light products. Use them to whip up delicious omelets.

Bacon

Sorry, but regular bacon is a red-light food. Acceptable alternatives are Canadian bacon and lean ham.

Dairy

Low-fat dairy products are a great source of protein in the morning. I always have a glass of skim milk with breakfast. Try moving down from 2% to 1% to skim in stages. I find that 2% tastes like cream now!

Low-fat or nonfat yogurts with sweetener and 1% or fat-free cottage cheese and cream cheese are also excellent sources of protein. Try to stay away from other cheeses, though, since they are generally high in saturated fat.

There are a wealth of delicious breakfast recipes in this book, from frittatas and omelets to homemade muesli and poached fruit. The breakfast recipes start on page 95.

"Your plan has turned off my inner demon's voice! I no longer crave sweet things. . . . I haven't had any chocolate in seven weeks (the longest I have been without it since birth, I swear!) and I am finding the plan easy to stick to and easy to manage. Now I know I am going to get down to a healthy body weight for the first time in my life."

—Sarah

WHAT TO HAVE FOR LUNCH

Since most of us spend the lunch hour away from home, either at work or at school, we tend to have two options for the midday meal: brown-bag it, or eat at a restaurant. In both cases, eating the green-light way is definitely doable—but there are some important guidelines to keep in mind.

Brown-Bagging It

This is really the best option for the G.I. Dieter. When you pack your own lunch, you can be sure that all the ingredients used are green-light. Here are some tips for turning your brown-bag into a green-light bag.

Sandwiches

This ever-popular lunchtime mainstay is usually high-G.I. and high-calorie. But there are several things you can do to make your sandwich green-light. First, use one slice of 100% stone-ground whole-wheat or other high-fiber bread. Spread on some mustard or hummus (no mayonnaise, butter, or margarine) and top with 4 ounces of lean deli ham, chicken, turkey, or fish. Add at least three vegetables, such as lettuce, tomato, onion, or green pepper. And

"I just started on this diet five weeks ago, and I love it! I am forty-three years old and have tried almost every diet out there. I even had my stomach stapled. BIG MISTAKE!!! Yesterday when I weighed in, I was 236 pounds. I started at 256 pounds. Twenty pounds! Usually two weeks is my limit, but I have no desire to quit now. Any diet I've been on is always such a chore. I am enjoying this so much, and my kids love the foods as well."

—Denise

do not top the sandwich with another slice of bread; simply eat it open-faced. Avoid egg-, chicken- and tuna-salad sandwiches that are made with fattening mayonnaise.

Salads

Salads are almost always green-light but are often short on protein. Add chickpeas or other types of beans, tuna, salmon, tofu, or 4 ounces of skinless, cooked chicken breast or other lean meat. Also watch the dressing. Use only low-fat and low-sugar versions. There are some great salad recipes starting on page 133.

Soups

In general, commercially canned soups have a relatively high G.I. rating because of the necessary high temperatures used in the canning process. There are a few green-light brands, such as Campbell's Healthy Request and Healthy Choice. Homemade soups made with green-light ingredients are the best option. Look at the recipes starting on page 116. Beware of all cream-based or pureed vegetable soups, since they are high in fat and heavily processed.

Pasta

The thing to watch out for here is quantity. Your pasta dish should contain only ¾ cup of cooked, whole-wheat pasta, as well as 1 cup of vegetables, ¼ cup of light pasta sauce, and 4 ounces of chicken or lean meat. But this still leaves you with dozens of delicious combinations.

Cottage Cheese, Fruit, and Nuts

A fast and easy lunch to take to work is cottage cheese and fruit. Pack 1 cup of fat-free or 1% cottage cheese, 1 cup of green-light fruit, and a handful of sliced almonds.

Dessert

Always have some fresh fruit for dessert. Pass on other sweet things.

Lunching Out

I have provided a handy removable page of tips for eating out at restaurants on page 315. At a sit-down restaurant, all you have to do is order an entrée that includes a low-fat source of protein, such as chicken or fish, and vegetables. Ask for extra vegetables in lieu of potatoes or rice, since restaurants tend to serve the red-light versions. Eating at a fast-food outlet, however, is another story. Because fast food is loaded with saturated fat and calories, with rarely a gram of fiber in sight, it is usually a good idea to avoid it. It's true that some major fast-food chains have recently started offering lower-fat options, but by going into the restaurant, you are walking into a den of temptation, surrounded by people scarfing down their usual fare of dietary disasters. If your alternatives are limited, however, here are some guidelines for navigating this gastronomic minefield.

Burgers

Dispose of the top of the bun and don't order cheese or bacon. Keep it as simple as possible. Grilled chicken is a better bet if it's available.

Fries

DON'T. A medium order of McDonald's fries contains 17 grams of fat (mostly saturated), about 50 percent of your total daily allowance.

Milkshakes

DON'T. The saturated fat and calorie levels are unbelievable.

Wraps

An increasingly popular alternative to the traditional sandwich is a wrap. Request a whole-wheat or low-carb tortilla or iceberg lettuce leaf, if available. If the wrap is made with pita bread, request whole wheat and ask that it be split in half so it's a single layer.

Submarines
One fast-food chain that should be applauded is Subway because of its extensive menu of low-fat sandwiches. Choose a 6-inch whole-wheat sub roll, top with turkey, ham, or chicken, plus lots of veggies, and eat your sub open-faced. Avoid cheese and mayonnaise unless they're low-fat. Do not be misled by the promotion of the Atkins-style wraps. They may be low-carb, but they are loaded with saturated fat. These recommendations apply to other similar sub shops too.

Fish or Shellfish
Both are excellent choices, provided there's no batter or breaded coating.

Chinese
My best advice is to steer clear of Chinese restaurants when trying to lose weight. The rice is a problem, because it is usually the high-G.I., glutinous kind that tends to stick together. The sauces, especially the sweet and sour ones, are high in sugar, and the noodles are also high-G.I.

WHAT TO SNACK ON

I can't stress enough how important it is to have three snacks every day. Snacks play a critical role between meals by giving you a boost when you most need it. Choose fruit, fat-free fruit yogurt with sweetener, cottage cheese, raw vegetables, nuts, or one of the snack recipes on pages 258 to 273. Watch out for other products that claim to be fat- and sugar-free, such as instant pudding. Unfortunately these products are usually made with highly processed grain (cornstarch) and are red-light. You might also want to look into food bars. Choose 50- to 65-gram bars that have around 200 calories each with 20 to 30 grams of carbohydrates, 12 to 15 grams of protein, and 5 grams of fat; Balance bars are a good choice. Many of the rest are high-G.I. and high-calorie, and contain lots of quick-fix carbs. Check labels carefully.

WHAT TO HAVE FOR DINNER

The typical North American dinner comprises three things: meat or fish; potato, pasta, or rice; and vegetables. Together, these foods provide an assortment of carbohydrates, proteins, and fats, along with other minerals and vitamins essential to our health.

Meat/Fish

Most meats contain saturated fat, so it's important to buy lean cuts and trim off all the visible fat. Chicken and turkey are excellent choices *provided all the skin is removed.* Fish and shellfish (not breaded) are also wonderful. In terms of quantity, the best measure for meat or fish is your palm. The portion should fit into the palm of your hand and be about as thick. Another good visual cue is a deck of cards.

Potatoes

The G.I. ratings of potatoes vary from high to moderate, depending on how they are cooked. Boiled new potatoes are the only kind you should eat, two or three at a sitting. Baked, mashed, and fried potatoes are all red-light.

Pasta

Though most pastas have a moderate G.I. rating and are low in fat, they have become a villain in weight control. That's because we tend to eat too much of it. Italians quite rightly view pasta as an appetizer or side dish, while North Americans make it a main course with sauce, cheese, and a few slivers of meat. Pasta should only make up a quarter of your meal (about ¾ cup cooked). Use whole-wheat or protein-enriched pasta, serve al dente (firm to the bite), and stay away from cream- and butter-based sauces.

Rice

Rice also has a broad G.I. range. The low-G.I. varieties are basmati, wild, brown, and long-grain because they each contain a starch, amylose, that breaks down more slowly than that of other rices. Serving size is critical, too. Allow ⅔ cup cooked rice per serving.

Vegetables/Salad

Eat green-light vegetables and salad to your heart's content. Serve two or three varieties of vegetables at every dinner as well as a salad.

Desserts

There is a broad range of low-G.I., low-calorie desserts that taste great and are good for you. Virtually any fruit qualifies, and there's always low-fat, no-sugar-added ice cream or frozen yogurt. And wait till you try the Baked Chocolate Mousse (page 301) and Pecan Brownies (page 287)!

Beverages

We all know that we are supposed to drink eight glasses of fluids per day. Personally, I find this a bit steep. But I do try to drink a glass of water before each meal and snack. Other than to stay hydrated, I do this for two reasons: One, having your stomach partly filled with liquid before the meal means you will feel full more quickly, thus reducing the temptation to overeat; two, you won't be tempted to wash down your food before it's been sufficiently chewed. The longer you take to eat, the less likely you are to overeat; it takes at least twenty minutes for the stomach to tell the brain it is full or satiated.

Water

Water is the best beverage choice because it doesn't contain any calories. Liquids don't seem to trip our satiety mechanisms, so it's a waste, really, to take in calories through them. Alcohol especially is a disaster for weight control because it is easily metabolized by the body, resulting in increased insulin production—so try to avoid it. It is also wise to stay away from fruit and vegetable juices, which we digest rapidly. If water is too boring for you, there are a number of no-cal or low-cal beverages to choose from.

Coffee

If you can, it's best to stick with decaffeinated coffee (see page 29). Never add sugar, and use only 1% or skim milk.

Tea

Both black and green teas have considerably less caffeine than coffee and also contain antioxidants that are beneficial to your heart health. Two cups of tea have the same amount of antioxidants as seven cups of orange juice or twenty cups of apple juice! So tea in moderation is fine, but use a sugar substitute if you normally add sugar, and 1% or skim milk. Herbal teas are also a good choice, though they do not contain the antioxidants that black and green teas have.

Soft Drinks

Most soft drinks are high in both sugar and caffeine, and are therefore red-light. Instead, opt for diet soft drinks that do not contain caffeine.

> "My mother, who is seventy-nine years young, was diagnosed with diabetes last spring and was a candidate for a heart attack. She was so afraid of having to take insulin every day that she was really motivated to follow your recommendations. She did so faithfully, and has lost 23 pounds! More importantly, her blood sugar has gone down to 4. As a daughter who cherishes her mom, I can't tell you how happy it makes me."
>
> —Monique

Skim Milk

Personally, my favorite beverage is skim milk. It's nonfat, and since most meals tend to be a bit protein deficient, drinking skim milk is a good way of making up for some of the shortfall.

Soy Milk

Soy milk can be an excellent choice, but buyer beware: Most soy beverages not only are high in fat, but also have added sugar. Look for soy milk that is nonfat or low-fat, has no flavoring (such as vanilla or chocolate), and has no added sugar.

For Vegetarians

If you are a non-meat eater and need to lose weight, the G.I. Diet is the program for you. All you have to do is continue to substitute vegetable protein for animal protein—something you've been doing all along. However, because most vegetable protein sources, such as beans, are encased in fiber, your digestive system may not be getting the maximum protein benefit. So try to add some easily digestible protein boosters like tofu and soy protein powder to your meals.

Okay, you now know exactly what, when, and how much to eat and drink to start shedding those pounds! In the next chapter, I'll outline the steps for getting started on the G.I. Diet.

chapter three

Getting Started in Phase I

The G.I. Diet consists of two phases, and the first, Phase I, is really the most exciting. This is the weight-loss portion of the diet, when you're putting your newly acquired knowledge into practice, developing healthier eating habits, trying new recipes, watching your waistline diminish, and feeling more energized. Once you have achieved your weight-loss goal, you enter Phase II—a heady moment. At that point all you'll have to do is maintain your new svelte frame, and perhaps buy some new clothes. Ready? Here are the essential first steps for launching yourself into Phase I.

STEP 1: SET THE GOAL

Before you do anything else, get your vital statistics on record. I can't think of a greater motivator than measuring your progress as the pounds drop off. Starting on page 318, you will find detachable log sheets to keep in the bathroom and record your weekly progress. Always weigh yourself at the same time of day, because a meal or bowel movement can throw off your weight by a couple of pounds. First thing in the morning, before you eat breakfast, is a good time.

Another measurement that is important to know is your waist circumference. It indicates your level of abdominal fat, which is significant to your health, especially your heart health. A woman's health is at risk if her waist circumference is 32 inches or more, and a man's is at risk if his is 37 inches or more. A measurement of 35 inches or more for women and 40 inches or more for men puts you in the high-risk category for heart attack and stroke. People with a high level of abdominal fat, whom doctors describe as apple-shaped, have a much greater chance of developing cardiovascular disease and Type 2 diabetes.

To measure your waist, take a measuring tape and wrap it around your natural waistline just above the navel. Don't be tempted to suck your stomach in! Just stand in a relaxed position and keep the measuring tape from cutting into your flesh. Now record your weight and waist measurement on the log sheet. I've added a Comments column so that you can also note how you're feeling, or any unusual events in the past week that might have some bearing on your progress. (Some readers have asked for additional log sheets. I suggest you photocopy some extra copies for future use before you start.)

Now that you know what your current weight and waist measurements are, you should set your weight-loss target. How much do you want to lose? The best method for determining this is the Body Mass Index, or BMI. It is the only internationally recognized standard for measuring body fat—which is the only part of you that we're interested in reducing. The BMI table on pages 42 to 43 is very simple to use. Just find your height in the left vertical column and go across the table until you reach your current weight, or the number closest to it. At the top of that column is your BMI, which is a pretty accurate estimate of the proportion of body fat you're carrying—unless you are under five feet, are elderly, or are overly muscled (and you really have to be a dedicated bodybuilder to qualify). If any of these characteristics apply to you, then these numbers, in all probability, do not.

BODY MASS INDEX (BMI)

BMI	normal						overweight					obese		
	19	20	21	**22**	23	24	25	26	27	28	29	30	31	32
height (inches)	body weight (pounds)													
58	91	96	100	**105**	110	115	119	124	129	134	138	143	148	153
59	94	99	104	**109**	114	119	124	128	133	138	143	148	153	158
60	97	102	107	**112**	118	123	128	133	138	143	148	153	158	163
61	100	106	111	**116**	122	127	132	137	143	148	153	158	164	169
62	104	109	115	**120**	126	131	136	142	147	153	158	164	169	175
63	107	113	118	**124**	130	135	141	146	152	158	163	169	175	180
64	110	116	122	**128**	134	140	145	151	157	163	169	174	180	186
65	114	120	126	**132**	138	144	150	156	162	168	174	180	186	192
66	118	124	130	**136**	142	148	155	161	167	173	179	186	192	198
67	121	127	134	**140**	146	153	159	166	172	178	185	191	198	204
68	125	131	138	**144**	151	158	164	171	177	184	190	197	203	210
69	128	135	142	**149**	155	162	169	176	182	189	196	203	209	216
70	132	139	146	**153**	160	167	174	181	188	195	202	209	216	222
71	136	143	150	**157**	165	172	179	186	193	200	208	215	222	229
72	140	147	154	**162**	169	177	184	191	199	206	213	221	228	235
73	144	151	159	**166**	174	182	189	197	204	212	219	227	235	242
74	148	155	163	**171**	179	186	194	202	210	218	225	233	241	249
75	152	160	168	**176**	184	192	200	208	216	224	232	240	248	256
76	156	164	172	**180**	189	197	205	213	221	230	238	246	254	263

Source: U.S. National Heart, Lung, and Blood Institute

						extreme obesity										
33	34	35	36	37	38	39	40	41	42	43	44	45	46	47	48	49
158	162	167	172	177	181	186	191	196	201	205	210	215	220	224	229	234
163	168	173	178	183	188	193	198	203	208	212	217	222	227	232	237	242
168	174	179	184	189	194	199	204	209	215	220	225	230	235	240	245	250
174	180	185	190	195	201	206	211	217	222	227	232	238	243	248	254	259
180	186	191	196	202	207	213	218	224	229	235	240	246	251	256	262	267
186	191	197	203	208	214	220	225	231	237	242	248	254	259	265	270	278
192	197	204	209	215	221	227	232	238	244	250	256	262	267	273	279	285
198	204	210	216	222	228	234	240	246	252	258	264	270	276	282	288	294
204	210	216	223	229	235	241	247	253	260	266	272	278	284	291	297	303
211	217	223	230	236	242	249	255	261	268	274	280	287	293	299	306	312
216	223	230	236	243	249	256	262	269	276	282	289	295	302	308	315	322
223	230	236	243	250	257	263	270	277	284	291	297	304	311	318	324	331
229	236	243	250	257	264	271	278	285	292	299	306	313	320	327	334	341
236	243	250	257	265	272	279	286	293	301	308	315	322	329	338	343	351
242	250	258	265	272	279	287	294	302	309	316	324	331	338	346	353	361
250	257	265	272	280	288	295	302	310	318	325	333	340	348	355	363	371
256	264	272	280	287	295	303	311	319	326	334	342	350	358	365	373	381
264	272	279	287	295	303	311	319	327	335	343	351	359	367	375	383	391
271	279	287	295	304	312	320	328	336	344	353	361	369	377	385	394	402

The ideal BMI is between 20 and 25. This range is quite generous, however, and your target BMI should be toward the lower end for women, toward the higher for men. BMI values under 18.5 are considered underweight, while those between 25.0 and 29.0 are classified as overweight. BMI values of 30.0 and over are considered obese. So put your finger on the BMI number 22 in the chart and drop down until you reach your height, which is shown in the left margin. The number at that intersection is what your weight should be to achieve that BMI target. Let's look at an example. If Sharon is 5 feet 6 inches and weighs 161 pounds, her BMI is 26, which is four notches above her target BMI of 22. This means that Sharon has to lose 25 pounds in order to bring her to her 22 BMI goal of 136 pounds.

If you are planning to lose up to 10% of your body weight, you should expect to lose an average of one pound per week. If you have more than 10% to lose, then you will lose more pounds per week. Typically someone with a BMI of over 30 will lose an average of two to three pounds a week. As a result, most people will take four to six months to hit their target. If that seems like a

"I heard some friends talking about your diet. I could tell they were losing weight successfully, and they were speaking very positively about it. So, I went out and borrowed the book from the library to see what all the fuss was about. I am 5 feet 3 inches and at that time I weighed 203 pounds and my waist was 42 inches. Today, I weigh 159 pounds and my waist is 32 inches . . . I have gone from size 18 pants to size 10 and from size XL in shirts to small or medium. I used to be able to shop only at clothing stores with larger sizes, but now I can shop wherever I choose."

—Karen

long time to you, think of it in terms of the rest of your life. What's less than half a year compared with the many, many years you'll spend afterward with a slim, healthy body? This isn't a fad diet—fad diets don't work. The G.I. Diet is a healthy, realistic, surefire route to permanent weight loss, and you can do it!

STEP 2: CLEAR OUT THE CUPBOARDS

At this point, your kitchen cupboard and refrigerator still probably contain some of the foods that are listed in the red-light column of the G.I. Diet Food Guide. Now how are you going to reach your goal with all this temptation at your fingertips? Give yourself a break and clear out your pantry, fridge, and freezer of all red- and yellow-light products. Throw them in the garbage, or better yet, donate the canned foods and other nonperishables to the local food bank and give the rest to neighbors, your children away at college, or anyone you know who doesn't happen to live in your house. This does not mean you will be depriving the nondieters in your family; this is a healthy way of eating for everyone. You're doing them a service!

STEP 3: GO SHOPPING

After you've enjoyed a good meal—and you're not remotely hungry—head over to the local grocery store and stock up on green-light foods. Before you go, you might also want to turn to the recipe section later in this book and pick out some new dishes to try. To make your first green-light shopping excursion simpler, I've included a detachable grocery list on page 313, which you can take with you. You will probably be buying more fruit and vegetables than usual, so be a little daring and try some varieties that are new to you.

I've tried to include a broad range of products in the G.I. Diet Food Guide, but of course I couldn't hope to include all the thousands of brands available in most supermarkets. Check labels when in doubt, and look for three things in particular:

1. Check the calorie content per serving—and make sure that the serving size is realistic. Some manufacturers will lowball the serving size in order to make the calories or fat content appear lower than that of their competitors' products.

2. Check the fat content, especially of saturated fat or trans fatty acids (often identified as "hydrogenated" fats), and look for a minimum ratio of 3 grams of poly- or mono-unsaturated fat to each gram of saturated fat. The total amount of fat should be less than 10 grams per serving.

3. Note the fiber content, since fibrous foods have a lower G.I. rating. Look for a minimum of 5 grams of fiber per serving.

STEP 4: START EATING THE GREEN-LIGHT WAY

Altering one's eating habits always requires some additional thought and preparation initially. As you begin to eat the green-light way, you will most likely have to consult the G.I. Diet Food Guide often. Before long, however, choosing the right foods will become second nature. To make starting the new plan as easy as possible, I suggest that you choose one or two standard breakfasts that you can eat every day for the first couple of weeks. This may sound boring, but you most likely do this now without thinking much about it. Perhaps you always have a bowl of cornflakes with fruit, or a toasted bagel with cream cheese. Decide what you are now going to have and give yourself enough time each morning to prepare and eat it. I myself look forward to starting each day with a bowl of oatmeal. I vary its flavor by adding different types of fruit yogurt or sliced fruit or berries. Perhaps you'd prefer a Yogurt Smoothie or a Canadian Bacon Omelet. You'll find these and many more breakfast ideas on pages 95 to 115.

While your dinner preparation routine is unlikely to change drastically, lunches and snacks, because they are often eaten away from home, will require some extra forethought. As I said earlier, you can eat the green-light way at restaurants, but your best option is to brown-bag it. Make any of the soups in the recipe section of this book ahead of time and store them in lunch-size quantities in the freezer. You could also prepare one of the salads on pages 133 to 165 the night before. Another suggestion would be to make extra when you are preparing dinner and have the leftovers for lunch the next day.

Be sure to plan out your snacks as well. Keep adequate supplies of ready-to-eat snacks such as fruit yogurt, cottage cheese, nutrition bars, fruit, and nuts at home, at work, in your purse, in your briefcase, and in the car. Bake other green-light snacks, such as Cranberry Cinnamon Bran Muffins, ahead of time and store them in the freezer. You can allow them to thaw in your lunch bag or defrost them in the microwave. A little advance preparation will ensure that you'll always have the right foods on hand when those

"I am a longtime believer that the most successful, wonderful things are simple and stand on their own merit without needing a lot of hype. This is what initially drew me to the G.I. Diet. I loved the way it was written, with such humility and common sense. I have been turned off again and again by diet books that spend more time promising success and sound like an infomercial than explaining the base of their diet philosophy. I started eating the G.I. Diet way 3 weeks ago. Can I tell you how tremendous I feel?"

—Maryellen

inevitable hunger pangs strike. Preparation will go a long way in guaranteeing your success on this diet.

STEP 5: ADD SOME EXERCISE TO YOUR ROUTINE

Dieting has a far greater impact on weight loss than exercise does. To give you some idea of how much exercise is required to lose just 1 pound of weight, have a look at the table below.

EFFORT REQUIRED TO LOSE 1 POUND OF FAT

	130-pound person	160-pound person
Walking (brisk; 4 mph)	53 miles/85 km	42 miles/67 km
Running (8 min/mile)	36 miles/58 km	29 miles/46 km
Cycling (12–4 mph)	96 miles/154 km	79 miles/126 km
Sex (moderate effort)	79 times	64 times

Clearly, an exercise regimen alone is not enough to reach your weight-loss goal (even if you are a sexual athlete!). However, exercise is an important factor in *maintaining* your desired weight. For example, if you were to walk briskly for a half hour every day for one year, you would burn up calories equaling 20 pounds of fat. Exercise increases your metabolism—the rate at which you burn up calories—even after you've finished exercising! It builds muscle mass as well, and the larger your muscles, the more energy (calories) they use. So start walking, bicycling, lifting weights, doing resistance exercises, and playing sports. Not only will it help your weight-loss efforts, it will dramatically reduce your risk of heart disease, stroke, diabetes, and osteoporosis.

These five steps will get you well on your way to achieving your weight-loss target.

Don't be surprised if you lose more than 1 pound per week during the first few weeks as your body adjusts to the new plan. Most of that initial weight will be water, not fat—remember, 70 percent of your body weight is water. Please don't worry if from time to time you "fall off the wagon." I probably live about 90 percent within the program and 10 percent outside it. It's important that you not feel as though you're living in a straitjacket. The fact is that I feel better and more energized when I stick to green-light foods, and you will too. Try to keep your lapses to a minimum; they will marginally delay your target date. Once you have reached your goal, you will be able to allow yourself more leeway in Phase II.

"This is the first time I have not felt hungry while trying to lose weight. There have been many *challenges, but your hints, especially about eating out, have made it so much easier. I keep apples, yogurt, and almonds at my two places of work and a Balance bar in my purse in case I miss a snack between jobs or if I get too busy."*

—Margie

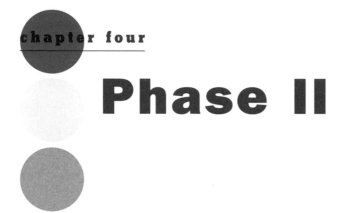

chapter four

Phase II

When you're ready to begin Phase II of the G.I. Diet, hearty congratulations are in order: You've reached your weight-loss target! You stuck to the principles of the program and are looking and feeling great as a result. All you have to do now is maintain your new weight. While this is definitely a less onerous phase than the first, maintenance can also be quite a challenge. In fact, those of you who have lost weight in the past only to regain it soon after may find the thought of Phase II a daunting prospect. I recently received an e-mail from a reader who lost 43 pounds in just six months on the G.I. Diet. Though she had reached her ideal BMI of 22, she was terrified of moving into Phase II because she feared gaining all that weight back. Statistics tell us that 95 percent of people who lose weight on a diet tend to put it back on. However, before you start feeling completely demoralized, please be aware that the primary reason for these bad odds is the diets themselves.

The truth is you can lose weight on virtually any diet. Yes, it may be bad for your health and you may be half-starving, but you will drop the pounds if you manage to stick to it. The problem is that almost all other diets—unlike the G.I. Diet—are completely unsustainable. And research tells us that there are three fundamental reasons why:

1. The diets require too much effort, asking dieters to count calories, carbs, or points and measure portions for every meal.

2. The diets leave people feeling hungry and deprived all the time and unwilling to continue.

3. The diets make people feel unwell because the regimens have a negative impact on their health. Many diets, if not most, are potentially damaging to one's health.

Clearly, it's pretty impossible to stick to a diet with any of the above characteristics. That's why I deliberately constructed the G.I. Diet to deal with each of those problems head-on. First, the program is simplicity itself. You will never again have to figure out the number of calories or carbs in everything you eat. It's all been done for you. If you can follow a traffic light, you can follow this diet. Second, if you eat all the recommended meals and snacks, you will not go hungry or feel deprived. This is the core reason why people are able to stick to this diet. Third, this program will not only do no harm to your health, it will actually improve it. Because the G.I. Diet includes whole grains, fruits and vegetables, low-fat dairy products, protein, and beneficial fats, it will actually improve your odds against today's major diseases, such as heart disease and stroke, diabetes, Alzheimer's, and many forms of cancer. In summary then, the G.I. Diet addresses and overcomes all the principal reasons why most diets don't work. And I guarantee that you will feel better on this diet than you ever have before.

This may be hard to believe, but when I reached my target weight after losing 22 pounds, I had to make a conscious effort to eat more in order to avoid losing more weight. My wife said I was entering "the gaunt zone"! In Phase II, you must eat more than you did during the weight-loss portion of the diet in order to maintain your new weight. Remember this equation: Food energy ingested must equal energy expended to keep weight stable. But I do have a few words of caution. For two reasons, you will require considerably fewer calories than you did before you started the diet. First, your body has become accustomed to doing with fewer calories and has to a certain extent adapted. Your body is more efficient than it was in the bad old days. Second, your slimmer body needs fewer calories to function. For example, if you lost 10 percent of your body weight, you now require 10 percent fewer calories.

The biggest mistake most people make when coming off a diet is to assume they can go back to eating the way they did before the diet. The reality is that you will probably need only a marginal increase in food energy to balance out the energy in–energy out equation. Only you can determine how big that increase should be. Try serving yourself slightly larger portion sizes or adding foods from the yellow-light category to your meals. Continue to monitor your weight each week, and if you start to gain, cut down a bit on the yellow-light foods; if you continue to lose, eat a bit more. If your weight remains stable, you've reached that magic balance and this is how you will eat for the rest of your life. You'll know what your body needs and you won't have to weigh yourself so often. You'll experience none of those hypoglycemic lows and will no longer crave junk food. And you'll be able to cheat once in a while without gaining any pounds. You will be in control of your weight.

SUPPLEMENTS

The G.I. Diet will provide you with the Recommended Daily Allowance (RDA) for most essential vitamins and minerals. The one possible exception is vitamin D. This is the true sunshine vitamin, not vitamin C as the Florida orange ads suggest. Though vitamin D is found in fatty fish and milk, which is supplemented with it, we depend primarily on sunshine to produce vitamin D in our bodies. Since many of us live in northern climes where sunshine is a scarce commodity in winter, and since we should all be lathered in sunscreen during the summer (protecting the skin but inhibiting vitamin D production), we are at risk for deficiency. Vitamin D is essential for the absorption of calcium for our bones. This is particularly of concern to women, especially post-menopause, in order to prevent osteoporosis.

The G.I. Diet's emphasis on low-fat dairy and fish will help, but it would be wise to take a multivitamin containing the recommended daily dosage of vitamin D, 400 IU.

PORTIONS AND SERVINGS

Here are some suggestions for how you might wish to modify your eating pattern in Phase II.

Breakfast

- Increase green-light cereal serving size; e.g., from ½ to ⅔ cup oatmeal.
- Add a slice of 100% whole-grain toast and a pat of margarine.
- Double up on the sliced almonds on cereals.
- Help yourself to an extra slice of Canadian bacon.
- Have a glass of juice now and then.

"I have lost 85 pounds in 22 weeks on the G.I. Diet, but the real news is what a difference that weight change has made to my appearance. I went to a family wedding last weekend and I was embarrassed by the attention I got. The room seemed to stop and gasp when I walked into the reception! I lost count of how many people asked what had happened, told me how good I looked, asked what diet I was on and how much weight I had lost. By the way, my cholesterol and other health stats are fantastic!"

—Derek

- Add one of the yellow-light fruits—a banana or a mango—to your cereal.
- Have a fully caffeinated coffee. Try to limit yourself to one a day, and make sure it's a good one.

Lunch

I suggest you continue to eat lunch as you did in Phase I. This is the one meal that contained some compromises in the weight-loss portion of the program because it is a meal that most of us buy each day.

Dinner

- Add another boiled new potato (from two or three to three or four).
- Increase the rice or pasta serving from ¾ to 1 cup.
- Have a 6-ounce steak instead of your regular 4-ounce.
- Eat a few more olives and nuts, but watch the serving size, as these are calorie heavyweights.
- Try a cob of sweet corn with a dab of nonhydrogenated margarine.
- Have a glass of red wine with dinner (see following page).
- Add an extra slice of whole-grain, high-fiber bread.
- Have a lean cut of lamb or pork (maximum 4-ounce serving).

Snacks

Warning: Strictly watch quantity or serving size.
- Have some light microwave or air-popped popcorn (maximum 2 cups).
- Snack on nuts, maximum ten.
- Indulge in a square or two of bittersweet chocolate (see following page).
- Eat a banana.
- Enjoy one scoop of low-fat ice cream or yogurt.

TREATS

Chocolate

This rich, luscious treat is the first thing all you chocoholics will want to incorporate back into your diet. And you can. Because chocolate contains large quantities of saturated fat and sugar, it is quite fattening. So choose chocolate with a high cocoa content (a minimum of 70 percent), because it delivers more chocoholic satisfaction per ounce, and have only a square or two every once in a while. Nibbled slowly or dissolved in the mouth, these two squares are all that's required to enjoy the taste and get the fix you need.

Alcohol

In Phase II, a daily glass of wine, preferably red and with dinner, is not only allowed, it's encouraged! Red wine is particularly rich in flavonoids, and when it is drunk in moderation (a glass a day), it has a demonstrable benefit in reducing the risk of heart attack and stroke.

What about beer? Well, unfortunately for all us beer aficionados, beer has an exceptionally high G.I. rating due to its malt content. Still, I do enjoy an occasional pint. Real discretion is required here, and if beer is that important to you, you are better off with the light or low-carb versions, which still have a high G.I. but are lower in calories. If you do drink alcohol, always have it with a meal. Food slows down the absorption of alcohol, thereby minimizing its impact.

With all these new options in Phase II, the temptation may be to overdo it. Remember to continue to weigh yourself weekly when you first begin in order to find your equilibrium. Once you do, eating the right amount will become second nature. You will find that Phase II is an easy and quite natural way to live, and that many of those high-fat foods you once thought you couldn't live without are no longer desirable.

Part Two
Living
the G.I. Diet

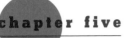

chapter five

Coach's Corner

By this point it's most likely safe to assume that you've committed yourself to the principles of the G.I. Diet and to losing weight permanently. Perhaps you've completed the five essential steps for getting started and have even begun to lose weight. Maybe you've already been on the diet for a few months and are seeing substantial results. Whatever stage you may have reached, you are bound to face the inevitable dieting hurdles that test everyone's firmest resolve. Food cravings, holidays and celebrations, vacations, and flagging enthusiasm are all challenges to our commitment to healthy eating. In this chapter I will give you some tips for dealing with these dietary hazards.

FOOD CRAVINGS

What makes losing weight particularly challenging is that we tend to enjoy and desire fattening foods such as chocolate, cookies, ice cream, peanut butter, chips, and so on. The most important thing to remember about cravings is that we're only human and it's natural to succumb to temptation every now and then. Don't feel guilty about it. If you "cheat," you aren't totally blowing your diet. You're simply experiencing a temporary blip in your good eating habits. If you have a small piece of chocolate cake after dinner, or perhaps a beer with the guys while watching the game, make sure you savor the extravagance by eating or drinking *slowly*. Really enjoy it. Then get back on track in the morning with a green-light breakfast and stick to the straight and narrow for the next couple of weeks. You will continue to lose weight, and that's what it's all about.

A friend of mine, who is a cardiologist, allows himself a few "red days" a month. These are days when he knows he has strayed from the guidelines of the G.I. Diet. To prevent red days from becoming a habit, he monitors them by marking them on his calendar, which is a great idea. And the G.I. Diet itself will help prevent lapses in two key ways. First, you will find that after you've been on the program for a few weeks, you will have developed a built-in warning system: You won't feel good physically when you eat a red-light food because your blood sugar will spike and crash. You'll feel bloated, uncomfortable, and lethargic, and you may even get a headache—a strong deterrent against straying into red-light territory. Second, because you are eating three meals and three snacks daily, you won't feel hungry between meals. If your stomach is too empty for too long, you will probably start longing for forbidden foods—so make sure you eat all the recommended meals and snacks every day.

Despite the diet's built-in security system, there will be times when a craving gets the better of you. What should you do? Well, you could try substituting a green-light food for the red-light food you're thinking about. If you want something sweet, try having fruit; applesauce; nonfat, sugar-free yogurt; low-fat ice cream with no added sugar; any of the green-light dessert recipes; a food bar; or a caffeine-free diet soft drink. If what you want is something salty and crunchy, try having a dill pickle or Dried Chickpeas (page 258). You could also make some Sage and Tomato White Bean Dip (page 259) and have it with celery sticks.

Your craving for chocolate in Phase I may be alleviated with a chocolate-flavored nutrition bar, with a light instant chocolate drink, or with Baked Chocolate Mousse (page 301) or Pecan Brownies (page 287). As you can see, there are many green-light versions of the foods we normally reach for when a craving strikes.

Sometimes, however, there isn't a likely substitute for the foods we miss. I have received many e-mails from readers who love peanut butter and say they cannot live without it. The thing to do here is to select the most nutritional product available—the natural kind that is made from peanuts only and has no additives such as sugar—and eat only a tablespoon of it once in a while. It's better to consume the good fats that are in peanuts than the red-light fillers that are found in other varieties of peanut butter. Don't be fooled into thinking that the "lite" versions are better for you. The amount of peanuts in these products has been reduced and sugar and starch fillers have been added. Remember that the more red-light foods you consume, the more you will slow your progress in achieving your target BMI.

HOLIDAYS AND CELEBRATIONS

We all know how much determination and gumption it takes to commit ourselves to a new weight-loss plan and how much drive it takes to clear one's cupboards, go shopping, and embark on an unfamiliar way of eating. That's why once we have managed to do all this, the last thing we want is for a holiday to come along and throw a wrench into our progress. Christmas, Thanksgiving, Easter, Passover, and so on all have one thing in common: an abundance of food. Holidays are generally centered around traditional feasts and dishes. But even so, you don't have to throw the G.I. guidelines out the window. You can stay in the green and still have a fun and festive holiday.

If you host the event yourself, you will be able to decide what type of food is served. Think of what you would normally eat during the holiday and look for green-light alternatives. For example, if you usually have a roast turkey with bread-based stuffing for

Thanksgiving, serve a roast turkey with wild or basmati rice stuffing instead. If you always make cranberry sauce with sugar, prepare it with a sugar substitute. My wife, Ruth, and I always add slivered almonds and chunks of orange to our cranberry sauce—delicious! There is no shortage of green-light vegetables to serve as side dishes, and dessert can be elegant poached pears or a pavlova with berries. You can put on a completely green-light feast without your guests even realizing.

If you celebrate the holidays at someone else's home, you will obviously have less control over the menu. You could help out the busy host by offering to bring a vegetable side dish or the dessert – a green-light one, of course. Once seated at the holiday table, survey the dishes and try to compose your plate as you would at home: vegetables on half the plate, rice or pasta on one quarter, and a source of protein on the other. Pass on the rolls and mashed potatoes; have extra vegetables instead. If you wish, you can allow yourself a concession by having a small serving of dessert. If you aren't particularly big on sweets, you might prefer to have a glass of wine instead. Try not to indulge in both.

Cocktail parties can also be fun, green-light occasions. Instead of alcohol, have a glass of mineral water with a twist of lime or lemon or a diet caffeine-free soft drink. If you really would like an alcoholic beverage, have only one and try to choose the least red-light option. Red wine is your best bet, or a white wine spritzer made with half wine and half sparkling water. Be sure to consume any alcohol with food to slow down the rate

"I don't see it as a diet, just a very fulfilling way of changing my eating habits for life. Many thanks, as I think I've finally found a diet that actually suits me and my lifestyle and actually works, and also occasionally lets me eat the things that I love."
—Annette

at which you metabolize it. Beer has a very high G.I. rating, so that's a real concession. Have one if you really want it, but make sure it's only one. Other alcoholic drinks are also high-G.I. and high-calorie.

If you host the cocktail party yourself, you can make all the appetizers green-light. Have a cooked, sliced turkey as a center-piece and offer lean sliced deli ham with a selection of mustards. Serve a variety of raw vegetables with a choice of low-fat dips and salsa. Hummus with wedges of whole-wheat pita, smoked salmon or caviar on cucumber slices, crab salad on snow peas, chicken or beef skewers, meatballs made with extra-lean ground beef, and sashimi with low-sodium soy sauce all make wonderful appetizers that everyone will enjoy. You can also provide bowls of nuts and olives, but remember to have only a few of each and don't linger nearby—it's too tempting to keep munching as you chat with your guests. Be sure to also serve a platter piled decoratively with a wide variety of green-light fruits.

If you are attending someone else's cocktail party, have a green-light meal before you go so you won't be tempted to eat too much. Then choose the low-G.I. appetizers and enjoy your time with friends and family.

VACATIONS AND DINING OUT

Going away on vacation usually means having to eat all your meals at restaurants—unless you spend a week at a cottage or a beach house where you can do the cooking yourself. It's not terribly diffi-cult, though, to put the G.I. guidelines into practice when dining out. First of all, you must ask the server not to leave the habitual basket of bread or rolls on your table. If it's not there, you won't be tempted.

Order a green salad to start and choose a low-fat dressing to be served on the side so that you can control the amount you use. Salads have a very low G.I. rating (if made with low-G.I.

ingredients) and will help to fill you up before the main course arrives, so you won't be tempted to overeat. Then order an entrée that includes a low-fat source of protein. Since boiled new potatoes are rarely available and you may not be sure what sort of rice is being served, ask for double the amount of vegetables instead. I've made this request in hundreds of restaurants and have never been refused. On page 315, I have included a detachable summary of dining-out and travel tips that you can keep in your wallet or purse.

When the server brings you the healthy, green-light meal you ordered, be sure to eat it slowly. There is a distinct connection between the speed at which we eat our food and feeling full or satiated. The stomach can take twenty to thirty minutes to let the brain know when it feels full. So you may be shoveling in more food than you require before your brain says stop. A friend of mine who is a physician noted that one of the common traits among his overweight physician colleagues was that they tended to bolt down their food. He thought that the habit probably stemmed from the days when they were busy residents and had to eat as quickly as they could in the hectic hospital environment. A movement in the eighteenth century advised chewing food thirty-two times before swallowing it! That's probably going overboard, but at least put your fork down between mouthfuls. If you savor your food by eating more slowly, you will leave the table feeling far more satisfied; you'll be amazed at the difference it makes.

Just because you are on vacation doesn't mean you shouldn't continue to eat three meals and three snacks daily. In your suitcase, pack some green-light snacks such as food bars, nuts, and any other nonperishables. Once there, you can buy nonfat, sugar-free yogurt; fruit; low-fat cottage cheese; and applesauce to snack on. Avoid the continental breakfasts offered in many hotels. They are generally made up of red-light foods and offer little in the way of nutrition. One option for breakfast is to buy your own fruit, green-light cereals, and milk at a supermarket and have breakfast in your hotel room.

If you are driving to your destination or are going on a road trip, your only option along the highway might be fast food. If you can, pack some green-light meals and snacks so you won't have to stop to eat. Otherwise, I have provided some tips for eating at fast-food outlets on pages 315 to 316.

STAYING MOTIVATED

Losing weight takes time and patience. If it took you five years to gain 20 pounds, how can you expect to lose them in the space of a month? Most people tend to lose the first few pounds very quickly. But as your body adjusts to the new way of eating, you might have a week during which you won't lose, while during other weeks you might lose 2 or 3 pounds. Remember that it's the average that counts, and you should target an average of *1 pound per week*. How do you stay motivated for the time it takes to reach your BMI target? Here are some good tips:

1. Maintain your weekly progress log. Success is a powerful motivator.

2. Set up a reward system. Buy yourself a small gift when you achieve a predetermined weight goal—perhaps a gift for every 3 pounds lost.

3. Identify family members or friends who will be your cheerleaders. Make them active participants in your plan. Even better, find a friend who will join the plan for mutual support.

4. Avoid acquaintances and haunts that may encourage your old behaviors.

5. Try adding what my wife, Ruth, calls a special "spa" day to your week—a day when you are especially good with your program. This will give you some extra credit in your weight-loss account to draw on when the inevitable relapse occurs.

6. Do not treat the G.I. Diet as a straitjacket. If you are on the program 90 percent of the time you are ahead of the game.

7. Keep a bag or backpack and for every 5 pounds you lose, add a few books to equal that weight. Then pick up the bag and carry it upstairs and back down. I guarantee that will be an absolute eye-opener and motivator. One reader built her bag up to 70 pounds and couldn't lift it and had to get a friend to help. The friend was so impressed that she started the G.I. Diet and has lost 30 pounds herself!

8. Check out **www.gidiet.com** to read about other dieters' experiences, to share your own, and to keep updated on new developments.

YOUR HEALTH

If your enthusiasm starts to flag, try to remember what you were thinking and feeling the day you decided to start the G.I. Diet. You were probably feeling fed up with the extra weight and wishing you were slim. You were probably concerned about your health, too. And you had good reason to be. The fatter you are, the more likely it is that you will suffer a heart attack or stroke, develop diabetes, and raise your risk for many cancers.

The two key factors linking heart disease and stroke to diet are cholesterol and hypertension (high blood pressure). High cholesterol is the key ingredient in the plaque that can build up in your arteries, eventually cutting off the supply of blood to your heart (causing heart attack) or your brain (leading to stroke). Hypertension puts more stress on the arterial system, causing it to age and deteriorate more rapidly, ultimately leading to arterial damage, blood clots, and heart attack or stroke. Excess weight has a major bearing on high blood pressure. In 2004 the American Physiological Society reported that hypertension is directly attributable to overweight and obesity in 75 percent of men and 65 percent of women.

Diabetes is the kissing cousin of heart disease in that more people die from heart complications arising from diabetes than from diabetes alone. And diabetes rates are skyrocketing: They are expected to double in the next ten years. The principal causes of the most common form of diabetes, Type 2, are obesity and lack of exercise, and the current epidemic is strongly correlated to the obesity trend.

Being overweight has also been linked to cancer. A recent global report by the American Institute for Cancer Research concluded that 30 to 40 percent of cancers are directly linked to dietary choices. Its key recommendation is that individuals choose a predominantly plant-based diet that includes a variety of vegetables, fruits, and whole grains—basically what the G.I. Diet recommends. So please do stick with it. Your weight has tremendous bearing on your health. What's worth more to you, a hamburger and fries or a long, healthy life to be shared with loved ones? I think the choice is obvious.

"I started the G.I. Diet at the beginning of March 2004 and was so excited to see the weight moving immediately! I was then motivated to start back using my treadmill, which I do now five days a week for forty minutes. This then inspired me to start doing light weights at the gym three days a week. It is now four months later, I'm 25 pounds lighter, and I feel stronger, have more energy, and am fitting into clothes I haven't worn in ages!"
—Alicia

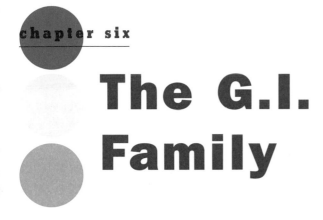

chapter six

The G.I. Family

As I mentioned in the previous chapter, one way of staying motivated on the G.I. Diet is to get a family member on board. If both of you are trying to lose weight together, you can support each other and have fun while doing so. More often than not, the letters I receive tell me about the results both husband and wife are seeing now that they're on the program together. But not everyone has someone in his or her family who wants or needs to lose weight. Does that mean they have to prepare separate meals for themselves? The answer is absolutely not.

The G.I. Diet is suitable for the whole family because it's really not a diet at all—it's a healthy way of eating, based on everyday foods. Phase II is the way we should eat throughout our entire lives.

Getting your partner or spouse eating the G.I. Diet way is important for several reasons. First, it's great to have mutual support and encouragement. Second, there's only one menu for shopping and cooking. Third, if you have children, then you both represent key role models for how to eat. "Do as I do" is a much more powerful motivator for children than "Do as I say, not as I do."

The best approach is to sit down and discuss with your partner your desire to change the way you eat. Point out that whether or not your partner needs to lose weight, making the change to the G.I. Diet is a healthier way of eating that will provide more energy and reduce the risk of stroke and major diseases such as diabetes, heart disease, and cancer, among others. Simply go to Phase II of the G.I. Diet for your partner if weight loss is not an issue, which means adding a few more choices to his or her menu and some adjustment to serving sizes.

If your partner is reluctant to change and give up those favorite red-light foods, then your best option is to introduce more green-light foods and provide him with tasty alternatives to red-light choices. This is exactly what many of the following recipes do: Take traditional meals and make them green-light. Easy-Bake Lasagna, Spaghetti and Meatballs, Vegetarian Shepherd's Pie, and Shrimp Caesar Salad are just a few examples. You will be amazed how quickly your partner will adapt. Not only do the green-light choices taste great, but by eating a more nutritional diet, your partner will actually feel better with more energy and no after-lunch slump.

For the stubborn objector, you have two choices. One, let your partner watch your transformation into a slimmer, more energetic, and healthier you. Others will comment on the change and ask you how you did it. Your partner will soon want to join you and emulate your success!

Alternatively, you can try the stealth method. Simply adjust the menu and say nothing. A friend of mine who went on the G.I. Diet began serving herself and her husband green-light meals for dinner every night without telling him they were based on the G.I. guidelines. He never even realized he was eating according to the recommendations of a diet plan until he had to have his pants taken in!

Phase II is also an ideal way for children to eat—and not just those who need to lose weight. We all know that the number of overweight and obese Americans has risen dramatically in the past several years due to poor eating habits and lack of physical activity. Unfortunately, being overweight has become all too common among children. In the United States the percentage of overweight has doubled in children and tripled in teenagers over the past twenty years. That's why it's so important to start introducing good eating habits to your children early on: It will serve them well in the future. Don't you wish you had never been introduced to junk food? If you had never tasted it, you wouldn't miss it now. If children don't get used to sugary soft drinks and candy, they won't develop cravings for these things later on.

Of course, this doesn't mean that your children shouldn't be allowed to enjoy their Halloween treats or birthday cake and ice cream. It's just that these things should be saved for special occasions. On the average day, children should eat a nutritious breakfast (not sugary cereals or Pop Tarts!), lunch, dinner, and snacks based on the G.I. guidelines. Fresh fruit, vegetables, fish, chicken, yogurt, whole-wheat bread, oatmeal, and apple bran muffins are all kid-friendly food. Just remember that growing children need sufficient fat in their diet—the good kind of fat found in fish, nuts, and vegetable oils.

We have found in our home that kids adapt easily to the G.I. way of eating. They like green-light foods and don't feel deprived. From the beginning, we made a point of serving our children healthy meals and snacks. We didn't keep soft drinks and other junk food in the house, but we didn't try to police our children either. Halloween always meant a period of "sugar shock," and birthday cakes were always thickly frosted. But the rest of the birthday party food we served was nutritious—sandwiches made with whole-wheat

> *"I am without a doubt a true believer in the G.I. way of eating (note I didn't say 'diet,' as it in no way resembles a diet, but a way of eating for a healthy life). After the first three days I felt fantastic . . . I didn't care whether I lost weight or not because I felt so good; weight loss was just an additional bonus."*
> —*Jenni*

food as comfort

Let's take a moment to acknowledge the important social and comforting role of food. From the minute we are held secure by our mothers and fed snug in their arms, food becomes connected with being held, being safe, and being comforted. And these connections stay with us for the rest of our lives.

As children we learn our eating habits and the importance of food from our parents. Often food is a reward for good behavior—ice cream, cookies, and candy are all used as treats. When we are ill as children we are fed our favorite foods so we will eat and get better. All our major celebrations, holidays, and activities include gathering together to eat. Sometimes we even eat to please our parents or to get their approval. All of this means that food can play a central role in feeling happy and content. For some people, who might be experiencing loneliness, anxiety, or high levels of stress, food can become a major source of comfort leading to overeating and spending down time snacking in front of the TV. For others, early behaviors have become habits so that the ritual of always having a snack when they came home from school now translates into walking in the front door and going directly to the kitchen for food.

Becoming aware of your eating behavior and habits is the first step toward changing them. So if this strikes a chord with you, take some time to examine your own eating behaviors and start trying to change those you are concerned about one at a time.

bread, vegetables with dips, and fruit—and loot bags contained little candy, if any. Our son David loved having oatmeal and yogurt for breakfast, although the consistency of it was always a matter of much negotiation: not too lumpy, not too smooth. We always tried to sit down for dinner as a family and catch up on what was happening with everyone. We never used dessert to bribe them to eat, and we usually served fruit for that course.

Our boys participated in making nutritious snacks. We have photos of the early muffin-makers complete with long aprons and large wooden spoons. They also enjoyed having raw vegetables for snacks if they were accompanied by interesting, low-fat dips. Now as adults, our sons continue to eat healthy diets and do not suffer from cravings for sweets or fast food. They love seafood, eat a wide variety of vegetables, and like to introduce their parents to new green-light foods. We first tried edamame (green soybean pods) at my eldest son's home.

So if you haven't yet done so, try serving all your family members green- and yellow-light meals. Don't tell them that they are following the G.I. Diet, just say that you'd like everyone to try eating a healthier way. The early experiences children have with food have tremendous impact on the way they will eat as adults.

"Last night, my partner Rod and I went to a dance and someone said that I looked 'hot.' You don't hear that every day at forty-seven! I was also able to dance to the Caribbean music all night. I figure I make a great date; I had one drink, no urge for the food provided, had an extended aerobic dance workout, and then could drive home. . . . Thanks again so much! I am having fun and feeling great."

—Karen

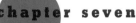

chapter seven

Frequently Asked Questions

Q. *Can I really eat as much of the green-light foods as I want?*

A. Yes you can, except where I recommend a specific serving or portion size. Serving sizes are important for green-light foods that have a higher G.I. rating or calorie content than others, such as pasta, rice, bread, nuts, and meat. Let common sense be your guide and keep everything in moderation. I wouldn't recommend eating twenty oranges a day, for example, or ten green-light muffins. That's going a bit overboard.

Q. *Is there any flexibility in this diet?*

A. Yes, but only you can determine which rules you can break and still lose weight. Many readers tell me they can't live without certain red-light foods such as regular coffee or peanut butter. If there's a product that is that important to you, go ahead and have it, but strictly limit the quantity you consume. Have only one cup of coffee or one tablespoon of peanut butter a day. One reader told me she was on the "Vegas" version of the G.I. Diet, meaning she had a glass of red wine every day on Phase I. She still lost 30 pounds and is wearing the same dress size she wore back in college.

Although you would lose weight faster if you followed all the guidelines of the G.I. Diet, it really is okay to commit only 90 percent to the program.

Q. *How is the G.I. Diet different from the Atkins Diet?*

A. The difference is like night and day. The Atkins Diet is based on high protein and animal fat (saturated fat) and low carbohydrates. The body, deprived of carbohydrates as its primary source of energy, is forced into a state of ketosis, which can cause serious long-term health issues such as osteoporosis and kidney damage. The high saturated fat content of the diet is associated with increased risk of heart disease, stroke, Alzheimer's, and prostate and colon cancers.

The G.I. Diet is quite the reverse. Carbohydrates such as fruit, vegetables, whole grains, beans, and low-fat dairy are all encouraged, not limited, while saturated fat is virtually eliminated—the perfect recipe for long-term good health.

Q. *Can I switch from Atkins to the G.I. Diet without gaining any weight?*

A. When you switch diets, you may see some temporary weight movement up or down for a couple of weeks as your body adjusts to a very different nutritional pattern. When things settle down you will be able to maintain your weight loss while giving your body the nutrition it needs for long-term health.

"I feel absolutely wonderful—I have energy to keep me going all day without having to nap—and my husband can't keep his hands off me! The doctor is stunned by my progress and is going to start recommending this diet to his other highly obese patients."
—Maeve

Q. *I thought aspartame and some other sugar substitutes were bad for your health. Why are you recommending them?*

A. A great deal of misinformation has been spread about sugar substitutes—driven mainly by the sugar lobby in the United States. All the major government and health agencies worldwide have approved the use of sweeteners and sugar substitutes and not a single peer-reviewed (scholarly) study has identified any health risks. For those who are still concerned about the safety of artificial sweeteners, there is a comprehensive rundown on sugar substitutes in the *U.S. Food and Drug Administration Consumer Magazine* (see www.fda.gov).

- Splenda (sucralose): Measures and tastes like sugar. Your best bet for both sweetening and baking.
- Sugar Twin/Sweet'n Low (saccharin): Some bitter aftertaste. Can be used for baking using a conversion chart.
- Sweet One (acesulfame-K): Also suitable for baking using a conversion chart.
- Equal (aspartame): Not suitable for baking. Some people are sensitive to aspartame.
- Stevia: Not FDA approved. One tablespoon of Stevia is equivalent to one cup of sugar.

Pregnant women should avoid these sugar substitutes, though in every other aspect the G.I. Diet is ideal for pregnant women.

"The big discovery for me was to find out how awful I feel when I go off your plan and start grabbing sweets or some such thing for a day. Y-U-C-K. I can't believe that I used to feel like that all the time before your book! I never would have thought that yogurt would become such a good friend."

—Bernice

Q. *Is the herbal sweetener Stevia a green-light product?*

A. Stevia is a South American herb that can be found in health-food stores. Although its popularity is growing, no long-term studies on its safety have been carried out—so I can't wholeheartedly recommend it. But so far it appears to be an acceptable alternative to sugar if used in moderation.

Q. *I understand that peanut butter has a low G.I. rating. If so, why is it red-light? Are the "lite" versions more acceptable?*

A. It's true that peanut butter has a low G.I. rating, but it is extremely high in fat and is dense in calories. Unfortunately, the "lite" varieties are even worse because the amount of peanuts has been reduced and sugar and starch fillers have been added to make up the shortfall. If you are going to "cheat" with an occasional tablespoon of peanut butter, make sure it's the natural kind that contains 100 percent peanuts and no added sugar.

Q. *Beans are listed as green-light, yet commercially canned black bean soup is red-light. Why?*

A. Beans are a classic green-light food, low in fat and high in protein and fiber. Commercially canned bean soups, however, are highly processed and therefore high-G.I. They are cooked at extremely high temperatures to prevent spoilage. This process breaks down both the outer protective skin of the beans and the starch granules inside—something that would normally be done by your digestive system. Because of this, canned black bean, split pea, and green pea soups are all high-G.I. Try one of the homemade bean soups instead, which are green-light and easy to make.

Q. *Dried apricots and cranberries are listed as yellow-light, yet they are used in some green-light recipes. Don't they raise the G.I. level of the recipes?*

A. Dried fruits actually have a low G.I. They are for the most part, however, high in calories, which is why most are listed in the red-light column. Dried apricots and cranberries have a lower calorie content, and the amount used in the recipes is so modest that they only marginally raise the calorie content, not enough to worry about.

Q. *I know you should avoid drinking alcohol in Phase I, but can you use wine in recipes?*

A. Absolutely! You can cook with wine even in Phase I. Adding a cup to a sauce that is going to serve four people means that each person will only be getting a quarter cup—much less than a full glass of wine. Also, much of the alcohol tends to evaporate in the cooking process.

Q. *Are low-calorie foods such as rice cakes or sugar-free Jell-O green-light foods?*

A. I'm afraid not. Although they don't have a lot of calories, they are digested quickly, leaving you looking for more food to keep your digestive system busy. Try to stick to green-light snacks, which are far more nutritious and satisfying.

Q. *What meat and poultry substitutes do you recommend?*

A. There are a number of meat substitute products available, and many of these products are green-light foods (you may also see them labeled as "meatless soy protein" or "textured vegetable protein" or "TVP"). Some of the most popular choices are burgers such as Boca and Yves, which are both high in protein and low in saturated fat. Check the fat levels of other products carefully. Avoid any breaded or battered versions.

Q. *I read that many high-fat foods such as premium ice cream are in fact low-G.I. Is this true?*

A. Yes it is. Fat acts as a brake on the digestive process, which means that fatty foods take longer to digest. But they are still red-light for two reasons. First, they are high in calories. Fat contains more than twice the calories per gram of protein or carbohydrates. Second, most high-fat foods contain saturated fats, which are bad for your health. Though the G.I. content of foods is a very important factor in determining whether a food is green-light or not, its calorie density and its impact on our health must also be taken into account. Saturated fat definitely has no place in the G.I. Diet.

Q. *I've been on the G.I. Diet for several weeks and have been very pleased with my progress, but now I seem to have hit a plateau. What should I do?*

A. Most people experience rapid weight loss during the first few weeks of the diet. That sets up the expectation that weight loss will continue at the same rate, but this is generally not the case. You should expect to lose an average of 1 pound per week. Don't be overly concerned if you hit a plateau. If you are following the G.I. Diet guidelines and are still above your recommended BMI, you will definitely reach your goal. If your plateau seems to be lasting a bit too long, think about what you have been eating lately and whether you may be straying a bit too far from the green-light column of the food guide. I received an e-mail from a reader who said he had reached a plateau and that his only indiscretion was a couple of peanut butter snacks a day. Well, the problem was that this "indiscretion" was delivering about 3,500 calories, or a pound of fat, to his waistline every week. No wonder he had hit a plateau!

For more information about the G.I. Diet, and to sign up for the free G.I. Diet Newsletter, visit my Web site at **www.gidiet.com**.

Part Three

Cooking the G.I. Way

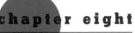

chapter eight

Introduction to G.I. Cooking

The notion of going on a diet can be a daunting one. People are often fearful that their food choices will be limited to unappetizing, bland, or difficult-to-prepare meals. Not so with the G.I. Diet! Just look at what's listed in the green-light column of the food guide, and you will see that there really is a wide-ranging variety of delicious foods. You can eat very well on the G.I. Diet and never have to sacrifice flavor or convenience. Not only are green-light foods high in fiber, low in saturated fat, and low in sugar, but they are some of the best tasting. Extra-virgin olive oil, for example, is rich in monounsaturated, or "best," fat and adds a wonderful, robust flavor to many dishes.

Good taste is always my first consideration when developing new recipes. I start with what I enjoy cooking and what my family and friends take pleasure in eating. I like to use plenty of fresh herbs, delicious spices, and ethnic flavors to come up with interesting and fun meals. In this collection, you will find some old favorites, like veal parmesan and beef fajitas, that I have modified to make green-light, as well as some new treats. By using less oil, avoiding white flour and sugar, and using cheeses for flavor enhancement only, you too can turn your own much-loved recipes into green-light dishes. My friend Emily Richards, one of the leading food writers of Canada; my wife, Ruth; our friends, and some readers who have written in to share recipes have all contributed to the selection of recipes here.

Cooking the G.I. way generally means cooking from scratch and avoiding heavily processed foods. But that doesn't mean you have to spend a lot of time in the kitchen. Most of the recipes in this book can be made in less than thirty minutes. I've included some breakfast recipes, such as Yogurt Smoothies and Muesli, for those mornings when you are on the run, as well as some recipes that are more suited for relaxing weekends, such as Light and Fluffy Pancakes and a Canadian Bacon Omelet. Any of the salad and soup recipes will form the basis of a satisfying lunch, and there are plenty of meatless, fish and seafood, poultry, and meat dishes to choose from for dinner. And because this isn't a deprivation diet but a new way of life, I've also included some recipes for desserts and snacks that I'm sure you will enjoy. I've tried all of them out on my family and friends and everyone has been amazed to discover that they are low-fat and low-G.I.—they taste that good. I hope that many of these green- and yellow-light dishes will become favorites among your own family and friends. Amid the recipes, I have included tips on ingredients, equipment, measuring, and side dishes, and I have given you a two-week menu plan to help you get started.

> *"I recently went home for Mother's Day, and my sister-in-law said, 'Dan, I find it so funny that before, you would eat like a bird. Now you say you are following a diet, but you haven't stopped eating.' She was right, and it is funny because I am losing weight and I feel great."*
>
> *—Dan*

INGREDIENTS

You will notice that not all of the ingredients in the recipes are strictly green-light. Occasionally I've added wine for depth of flavor, as well as small amounts of sauces that contain sugar, and dried fruit. This doesn't mean that the recipe is yellow- or red-light. The quantities are so minor that they will have little to no effect on your blood sugar level. Don't feel that you have to omit them to stay in the green.

To replace sugar in recipes, I've had great success with Splenda and have found the flavor quite good. Look for the granular type that comes in boxes because it is the easiest to use; you can measure out the amount just like sugar.

EQUIPMENT

Nonstick skillets

When cooking low-fat dishes, it's useful to have a few nonstick skillets on hand in various sizes. You only need a minimal amount of oil when using them (sometimes none at all), and food slides right off the pan. Remember that the recommended cooking heat for nonstick surfaces is no higher than medium-high and that you should use nonabrasive utensils and brushes only. Wash your skillet with hot soapy water and a nylon brush; do not put it in the dishwasher, which will damage the nonstick coating. If your pans show signs of wear, consider buying new ones for better performance.

Grill pans and indoor grills

The tips I gave above for caring for your nonstick pans also apply to grill pans and indoor grills. When using them, you only need a light brush or spray of oil. A grill pan keeps the food you are cooking out of the fat and gives that grilled look when you don't have an outdoor barbecue.

Pots and pans

Ever wondered what the difference is between a pot and a pan? Well, a pot usually has two handles and a pan has only one. They can pretty much be used interchangeably. A Dutch oven is just a large pan or pot that has a lid—most people have one without even realizing it!

MEASURING

To ensure success with these recipes, be sure to use measuring cups and spoons. Use wet measuring cups, which are usually glass or plastic and have a pouring spout, to measure milk, juice, stock, and water. Look at the wet ingredients at eye level on a flat surface for correct measurements. Use dry measuring cups, which are plastic or metal and nest inside each other, to measure flour, sugar, pasta, and anything with a thick consistency like yogurt and margarine. Dry ingredients are measured by spooning into the measuring cup and leveling it off with the back of a knife without tapping or adding more. Measuring spoons are usually metal or plastic and can be used for both wet and dry ingredients. You should also level off measuring spoons with a flat surface.

A kitchen scale can be very useful when weighing pasta, meat, vegetables, and fruit. Look for one with a bowl or container on top for ease of measuring. If you don't have a scale and you'd like to

"I wanted to let you know that I fit into a gown that I bought last January on sale. At the time, it was a bit too small on me. Now, the store has had to take it in for me. I was at a wedding last Saturday and one of my aunts said that I looked like a movie star. One of my cousins did a double take when she realized that it was me!! I cannot thank you enough."

—Bobbi

measure out 6 ounces of long pasta—which is what I've used in the recipes in this book—simply grab a handful of spaghetti or linguine tightly and squeeze into a bundle. It should measure 1 inch across.

SIDE DISHES

Almost all of the dinner recipes I have included in this book should be accompanied by side dishes. A quarter of your plate should be filled with a starchy carbohydrate such as pasta, rice, or boiled new potatoes. Since overcooking tends to raise the G.I. level of food, boil pasta until it is just al dente, or still firm when bitten, and take rice off the heat before it starts to clump together. Small new potatoes will only take about ten minutes to boil or steam.

Half your plate should be filled with green-light vegetables and salad. Again, do not overcook the veggies; they should be tender-crisp. Most people I know are not avid fans of mushy, flavorless vegetables anyway. See pages 274 to 277 for recipes for side vegetables.

"About 6 weeks ago, I had an epiphany: If I didn't lose weight, I was going to be the third person in my family to eat themselves into diabetes. I had ballooned to 260 pounds of pure blubber at the ripe old age of twenty-two. . . . I have been following the G.I. Diet nearly 100 percent for 6 weeks now, along with an hour of cardio a day, and have lost a little over 2 pounds every week. I am never hungry and never lacking energy. Now both my parents have bought the book and are following accordingly."
—Kyle

SAMPLE TWO-WEEK MEAL PLAN

Use this meal plan as a guide. Substitute different kinds of fruit, yogurts, omelets, healthy soups, snacks, and so on to provide variety. Remember to drink 6 to 8 glasses of water a day.

DAY ONE

Breakfast	Muesli (page 96)
Snack	Cranberry Cinnamon Bran Muffin (page 266)
Lunch	Mushroom, Barley, and Beef Soup (page 129)
	Open-face turkey sandwich with Sage and Tomato White Bean Dip (page 259)
	Carrot and celery sticks
Snack	Orange and nonfat fruit-flavored yogurt with sweetener
Dinner	Hunter-Style Chicken (page 214)
	Long-grain rice and asparagus
Snack	Basmati Rice Pudding with Peaches (page 298)

DAY TWO

Breakfast	Homey Oatmeal (page 98)
	Grapefruit sections with 1% cottage cheese
Snack	Cranberry Cinnamon Bran Muffin (page 266)
Lunch	Tuscan White Bean Soup (page 121)
	Grilled Chicken Salad (page 152)
	½ whole-wheat pita

Snack	Apple and 1% cottage cheese
Dinner	Almond Haddock Fillets (page 196) Baby carrots and long-grain rice Zucchini Salad (page 138)
Snack	Apple Pie Cookie (page 285) Glass of skim milk

DAY THREE

Breakfast	Canadian Bacon Omelet (page 107) Slice of 100% stone-ground whole-wheat toast Tomato wedges
Snack	Whole-Wheat Scone (page 263) Orange
Lunch	Lemon Dill Lentil Salad (page 146) Open-face ham sandwich with Roasted Red Pepper Hummus (page 260) Pickle
Snack	Apple Pie Cookie (page 285) Glass of skim milk
Dinner	Asian Greens and Tofu Stir-Fry (page 174) with basmati rice Green salad
Snack	Fresh Fruit Bowl (page 273) with 2 to 3 tablespoons nonfat sour cream

DAY FOUR

Breakfast	Muesli (page 96) Canadian bacon Slice of 100% stone-ground whole-wheat toast Sliced peach

| Snack | Whole-Wheat Scone (page 263) |
| | Apple |

Lunch	Ham and Lentil Soup (page 128)
	Tangy Red and Green Coleslaw (page 137)
	½ whole-wheat pita

| Snack | Roasted Red Pepper Hummus (page 260) with baby carrots, broccoli, and cucumber |

| Dinner | Horseradish Burger (page 227) |
| | Mediterranean Bean Salad (page 143) |

| Snack | Pecan Brownie (page 287) |
| | Glass of skim milk |

DAY FIVE

Breakfast	Cinnamon French Toast (page 102)
	Sliced ham
	Orange

| Snack | Almond Bran Haystack (page 271) |
| | Glass of skim milk |

| Lunch | Crab Salad in Tomato Shells (page 156) |
| | 1% cottage cheese with applesauce |

| Snack | Peach and nonfat fruit-flavored yogurt with sweetener |

Dinner	Veal with Fennel and Mushrooms (page 245)
	Spaghetti
	Steamed baby carrots
	Tomato, Zucchini, and Wheat Berry Salad (page 144)

| Snack | Berry Crumble (page 299) |

DAY SIX

Breakfast	Puffy Baked Apple Pancake (page 105) Canadian bacon
Snack	Almond Bran Haystack (page 271) Glass of skim milk
Lunch	Steak Salad with Peppers and Tomatoes (page 160)
Snack	Tofu pudding
Dinner	Easy-Bake Lasagna (page 180) Tossed salad
Snack	Poached Pears (page 297) with Sweet Yogurt Cheese (page 279)

DAY SEVEN

Breakfast	Morning Glory Poached Fruit (page 97) Florentine Frittata (page 106) Slice of 100% stone-ground whole-wheat toast
Snack	Nonfat fruit-flavored yogurt with sweetener
Lunch	Avocado and Fresh Fruit Salad (page 142) Open-Face Chicken Reuben Sandwich (page 224) with Roasted Red Pepper Hummus (page 260)
Snack	Dried Chickpeas (page 258)
Dinner	Salmon Steaks with Light Dill Tartar Sauce (page 199) Green beans and new potatoes Creamy Cucumber Salad (page 136)
Snack	Glazed Apple Tart (page 300)

DAY EIGHT

Breakfast	Homey Oatmeal (page 98) with yogurt, nuts, and fruit Tea or decaf coffee
Snack	Cranberry Cinnamon Bran Muffin (page 266)
Lunch	Open-Face Chicken Reuben Sandwich (page 224) Small Green Salad with Vinaigrette (page 133) Glass of skim milk
Snack	1% cottage cheese with orange sections and a few almonds
Dinner	Classic Meat Lasagna (page 240) Green Salad with Vinaigrette (page 133) Frozen Blueberry Treat (page 293)
Snack	Dried Chickpeas (page 258)

DAY NINE

Breakfast	Muesli (page 96) with fruit yogurt Orange Tea or decaf coffee
Snack	2 Chocolate Almond Slices (page 284) Pear slices
Lunch	Cauliflower and Chickpea Soup (page 122) ½ whole-wheat pita with canned salmon, tomato, and lettuce
Snack	Laughing Cow low-fat cheese with celery, carrots, and cherry tomato
Dinner	Chicken Jambalaya (page 217) Basmati rice

Green Salad with Vinaigrette (page 133)

Berries and yogurt

| Snack | 2 Oatmeal Cookies (page 280) |
| | Glass of skim milk |

DAY TEN

Breakfast	Florentine Frittata (page 106)
	1 slice whole-grain toast
	Tea or decaf coffee

| Snack | 1% cottage cheese with fresh fruit and almonds |

| Lunch | Niçoise Salad (page 151) |
| | ½ whole-wheat pita |

| Snack | Over-the-Top Bran Muffin with Pears (page 261) |

Dinner	Hunter-Style Chicken (page 214)
	White Bean Mash (page 275)
	Broccoli and tomato wedges

| Snack | 2 Chocolate Drop Cookies (page 283) |
| | Glass of skim milk |

DAY ELEVEN

Breakfast	Homey Oatmeal (page 98)
	Orange
	Tea or decaf coffee

Snack	Oatcake (page 272)
	Fruit
	½ glass of skim milk

Lunch	Southwest Omelet Roll-Up (page 110) 1 slice whole-wheat bread Fruit salad
Snack	Laughing Cow cheese with 2 high-fiber crisp breads
Dinner	Sloppy Joes (page 239) ½ whole-wheat pita Roasted Red Pepper Hummus (page 260) with cucumber, broccoli, and bell pepper slices
Snack	2 Blueberry Bars (page 270) ½ glass of skim milk

DAY TWELVE

Breakfast	Muesli (page 96) with fresh fruit and almonds Tea or decaf coffee
Snack	Over-the-Top Bran Muffin with Pears (page 261)
Lunch	Arugula and Roasted Pepper Pasta Salad (page 140) Chopped cooked chicken breast Fresh fruit
Snack	Boursin light cheese with tomato slices and 1 high-fiber crisp bread
Dinner	Pan-Seared White Fish with Mandarin Salsa (page 206) Green beans and mixed rice Green Salad with Vinaigrette (page 133)
Snack	1 Chocolate Almond Slice (page 284) Glass of skim milk

DAY THIRTEEN

Breakfast	Buttermilk Pancakes (page 101) Fresh berries Tea or decaf coffee
Snack	Low-fat fruit yogurt with sweetener, sprinkled with bran buds
Lunch	Shrimp Caesar Salad (page 158) 1 slice whole-wheat bread
Snack	Apple and a few almonds
Dinner	Steak Fettuccine (page 230) Green Salad with Vinaigrette (page 133) Fruit-Filled Pavlova (page 294)
Snack	Oatmeal Cookie (page 280) Glass of skim milk

DAY FOURTEEN

Breakfast	Cinammon French Toast (page 102) Canadian bacon Sliced strawberries Tea or decaf coffee
Snack	Laughing Cow low-fat cheese 1 high-fiber crisp bread 1 pear
Lunch	Cauliflower and Chickpea Soup (page 122) Open-face sandwich with lean deli ham on whole-grain bread with tomato slices, lettuce, cucumber, and mustard

Snack	1 tablespoon Roasted Red Pepper Hummus (page 260) with cucumber and baby carrots
Dinner	Quick Fish Steak with Tomato Chickpea Relish (page 194)
	Basmati rice and green beans
	Green Salad with Vinaigrette (page 133)
	Almond-Crusted Pears (page 292)
Snack	Nonfat fruit-flavored yogurt sprinkled with bran buds

"As a grade-six teacher, I used to feel like I would 'hit a wall' at about one-thirty or two o'clock every afternoon, but now that my blood sugar levels are more consistent, I feel fine throughout the afternoon. I always have a food bar handy in my desk in case I feel a little hungry. I guess the best thing has been that I don't feel deprived or that I'm on a diet; rather, I feel I'm just eating better."

—Mary

chapter nine

The
Recipes

The G.I. Diet is a program of abundance. The foods you can eat on it are varied and flavorful. Here are my family's favorite green-light recipes. You will find delicious versions of your family's favorite foods, like lasagna, pizza, and sloppy joes, as well as things that you may not cook all the time, like simple frittatas, soups, and casseroles. Plus there are recipes for special occasions, dinner parties, and for times when you just want to try something different. A few recipes are yellow-light for when you shift into Phase II. For vegetarians, I have included a section of meatless main dishes as well as vegetarian options for many of the other recipes. Before my middle son became a vegetarian in his teens, I rarely had a meatless meal. Now my family frequently eats delicious vegetarian dinners.

Though the recipes are divided into sections, I encourage you to be flexible. Many breakfast dishes make great lunch or brunch dishes. Most salads are terrific for lunch or dinner. Most snacks and many desserts are interchangeable as I have indicated in the fourteen-day meal planner on pages 85–93.

One final note: The recipes usually call for low-fat mayo, sour cream, or yogurt. If you are able to find a fat-free variety, use that instead.

Bon appétit!

BREAKFAST

Yogurt Smoothies ●

2 servings

You don't need a blender to make these fruit-flavored smoothies—a simple whisk will do. But if you prefer a very frothy smoothie, by all means use a blender.

> *2 cups skim milk*
> *1 container (6 ounces) nonfat fruit-flavored yogurt*
>   *with sweetener*
> *½ teaspoon sugar substitute*

In a small bowl, whisk together the milk, yogurt, and sugar substitute until smooth.

Options:

Thicker smoothies: Break out the blender and add 1 cup hulled, sliced strawberries or raspberries.

Dessert smoothies: Use 1 cup of low-fat, no-added-sugar ice cream instead of the yogurt and buzz up with the milk, omitting the sugar substitute.

Muesli ●

Makes 3 1/2 cups

My friend Lesleigh introduced me to this delicious and healthy start to the day. Eat it with skim milk or yogurt (see Hint).

> 2 cups old-fashioned rolled oats 8
> ¾ cup oat bran 3
> ¾ cup sliced almonds 3
> ½ cup shelled unsalted sunflower seeds 2
> 2 tablespoons wheat germ ×   100 grams
> ¼ teaspoon ground cinnamon 1

In a large resealable plastic bag, combine the oats, oat bran, almonds, sunflower seeds, wheat germ, and cinnamon. Use a rolling pin to crush the mixture into coarse crumbs. Shake the bag to combine the mixture.

Storage:
Keep the dry mix in a resealable bag or airtight container at room temperature for up to 1 month.

Helpful Hint:
If you like, prepare your muesli the traditional Swiss way: The night before, combine ⅓ cup of the muesli with ⅓ cup of skim milk or water, cover, and refrigerate. Then in the morning, combine the mixture with one 6-ounce container of nonfat fruit yogurt with sweetener. Enjoy it cold, or pop it in the microwave for a hot breakfast.

632.93 Calories
34.77 Protein
62.10 Carbs
35.32 Fat

Morning Glory Poached Fruit ●

4 servings

I f you don't have time to eat breakfast at home, make this fruit the
night before or a few days before and take it with you. It also
makes a wonderful mid-morning or mid-afternoon snack.

2 cups water
2 cinnamon sticks, broken in half
4 thin (coin-sized) slices peeled fresh ginger
3 tablespoons sugar substitute
2 apples, cored and coarsely chopped
2 pears, cored and coarsely chopped
1 grapefruit
1 orange
2 cups fat-free or 1% cottage cheese or
  Yogurt Cheese (page 279)

1. Place the water, cinnamon sticks, ginger, and sugar substitute in
a small saucepan and bring to a boil. Reduce the heat, add the
apples and pears, and simmer until tender-crisp, about 5 minutes.
Remove the fruit with a slotted spoon to a large bowl, reserving the
syrup. Let cool.

2. Meanwhile, using a serrated knife, cut off both ends of the
grapefruit. Starting at one end, cut the skin and white pith off the
grapefruit, leaving the fruit intact. Repeat with the orange. Using
the same knife, cut segments between membranes of the grapefruit
and orange and add, along with their juices, to the bowl with the
apples and pears. Serve with cottage cheese and drizzle with some
of the cinnamon syrup, if desired.

Homey Oatmeal ●

4 servings

This hot breakfast is guaranteed to keep you feeling satisfied all morning. You can vary the flavor by topping it with fresh fruit such as berries or chopped apple.

2 cups skim milk
1½ cups water
¾ teaspoon ground cinnamon
½ teaspoon salt
1⅓ cups old-fashioned rolled oats
¼ cup wheat germ
¼ cup chopped almonds
3 tablespoons sugar substitute

Place the milk, water, cinnamon, and salt in a large saucepan and bring to a boil. Stir in the oats and wheat germ and return to a boil. Reduce the heat to low and cook, stirring, until thickened, about 8 minutes. Stir in the almonds and sugar substitute.

Wheat Berry Breakfast ●

3 servings

This recipe comes from G.I. dieter Gwyneth, who has been making it for many years—especially during canoe trips. You can buy wheat berries, also known as soft or hard wheat kernels, at health or bulk food stores. Covering them with water, and soaking overnight allows them to crack open, producing a delicate kernel of wheat.

> *1 cup wheat berries*
> *4 cups water*
> *Skim milk*
> *Sugar substitute*
> *Sliced almonds*
> *Fresh fruit (such as berries or peaches)*

1. Place the wheat berries and water in a large saucepan and bring to a boil. Reduce the heat and simmer, uncovered, for 20 minutes.

2. Place the wheat berries with their cooking water in a large thermos, Mason jar, or heat-proof airtight container, and seal tightly. Let stand overnight. (If you have no thermos, you may keep the wheat berries and their cooking water in the saucepan, cover it, and refrigerate overnight.)

3. Drain any water from the wheat berries. Serve about ¾ cup of berries with milk, sugar substitute, almonds, and fruit as desired.

Storage:
If there are any leftovers, be sure to refrigerate them.

Light and Fluffy Pancakes ●

16 pancakes; 4 to 6 servings

Pancakes make weekend mornings special. You can also enjoy them during the work week by making and freezing them ahead of time. When Tuesday or Wednesday rolls around, simply pop the frozen pancakes into your toaster or microwave and enjoy.

1¼ cups all-purpose flour
¾ cup whole-wheat flour
¼ cup wheat bran
1 tablespoon baking powder
¼ teaspoon salt
¼ teaspoon ground nutmeg
1½ cups skim milk
½ cup liquid egg
2 tablespoons canola oil
2 tablespoons sugar substitute
1 teaspoon vanilla

1. Combine the all-purpose and whole-wheat flours, bran, baking powder, salt, and nutmeg in a large bowl. In another bowl, whisk together the milk, liquid egg, oil, sugar substitute, and vanilla. Pour the milk mixture over the flour mixture and whisk until smooth.

2. Heat a nonstick griddle or large nonstick skillet over medium heat. Ladle about ¼ cup of batter onto the griddle for each pancake. Cook the pancakes until bubbles appear on top, about 2 minutes.

3. Using a spatula, flip the pancakes and cook for another minute or until golden. Transfer to a plate and cover to keep warm. Repeat with the remaining batter.

Storage:

These pancakes can be frozen in a single layer on a baking sheet until firm. Place them in an airtight container once frozen.

Buttermilk Pancakes ●

16 pancakes; 4 to 6 servings

This recipe comes from Michelle R. Though buttermilk might sound as though it's rich and indulgent, it actually is low in fat and adds a wonderful tang to these pancakes. For a delicious topping, serve with berries or sliced peaches and a spoonful of fat-free sour cream. If you like your sour cream sweet, blend in a small amount of brown sugar substitute sweetener.

> *2 cups whole-wheat flour*
> *1 tablespoon baking powder*
> *2 teaspoons sugar substitute*
> *2 cups buttermilk*
> *⅓ cup liquid egg*
> *2 tablespoons canola oil*
> *1½ teaspoons vanilla*

1. Combine the flour, baking powder, and sugar substitute in a large bowl. In another bowl, whisk together the buttermilk, liquid egg, oil, and vanilla. Pour the buttermilk mixture over the flour mixture and whisk until smooth. You may store the batter, covered, in the fridge overnight for use the next day if you like.

2. Heat a nonstick griddle or large nonstick skillet over medium heat. Ladle about ¼ cup of batter onto the griddle for each pancake. Cook until bubbles appear on top, about 2 minutes.

3. Using a spatula, flip the pancakes and cook for another minute, or until golden. Transfer to a plate and cover to keep warm. Repeat with the remaining batter.

Cinnamon French Toast ●

2 servings

S erve this family favorite with slices of ham or Canadian bacon and extra strawberries for a complete breakfast.

> ¾ cup liquid egg
> ½ cup skim milk
> 1 tablespoon sugar substitute
> 1 teaspoon vanilla
> ½ teaspoon ground cinnamon
> Pinch of salt
> 4 slices stone-ground whole-wheat bread
> 1 teaspoon canola oil
> 2 cups sliced strawberries
> ½ cup nonfat fruit-flavored yogurt with sweetener

1. Whisk together the liquid egg, milk, sugar substitute, vanilla, cinnamon, and salt in a shallow dish. Dip each slice of bread into the egg mixture, making sure to coat both sides.

2. Meanwhile, brush the oil onto a nonstick griddle or large nonstick skillet and heat over medium-high heat. Cook the bread, turning once, until golden brown on both sides, about 4 minutes total. Serve with strawberries and yogurt.

Berry Crêpes ●

10 crepes; 4 servings

Crêpes may sound difficult to make, but they are actually quite simple. Just make sure the pan is hot when you add the crêpe batter. The batter should start to set as soon as you swirl it around in the pan.

> ½ cup whole-wheat flour
> 1 tablespoon ground flax seed or wheat germ
> Pinch of salt
> 1 cup skim milk
> ½ cup liquid egg
> 1 teaspoon vanilla
> 1 teaspoon canola oil
> 2 cups fresh blueberries
> 2 cups fresh raspberries
> 2 tablespoons sugar substitute
> 1 tablespoon chopped fresh mint (optional)
> Pinch of ground cinnamon
> 1 cup Yogurt Cheese (page 279)

1. Combine the flour, flax seed, and salt in a medium bowl. In another bowl, whisk together the milk, liquid egg, and vanilla. Pour the liquid mixture over the flour mixture and whisk until smooth. Let the batter stand at room temperature for at least 15 minutes, or cover and refrigerate for up to 2 hours.

2. Brush a small nonstick or crêpe pan with just enough oil to lightly coat it. Heat the pan over medium heat. Pour in a scant ¼ cup of the batter, swirling the pan to cover the bottom. Cook the crêpe until firm and slightly golden, about 2 minutes. Flip the crêpe and cook

(continued)

on the other side for another 30 seconds. Remove to a plate and cover to keep warm. Repeat with the remaining batter (see Note).

3. Combine the blueberries, raspberries, sugar substitute, mint (if using), and cinnamon. Put about ⅓ cup of the berry mixture in the center of each crêpe and roll up. Serve with Yogurt Cheese and the remaining berries.

Note:
Sometimes the first crêpe doesn't work out, so the recipe gives you a bit of extra batter for practice. If you're a pro at it, you'll have a crêpe to snack on while you cook the rest.

Puffy Baked Apple Pancake ●

4 servings

Y ou can replace the apple in this recipe with your favorite seasonal fruit. Try peaches or pears.

>*4 cooking apples, cored*
>*2 teaspoons nonhydrogenated soft margarine*
>*⅓ cup apple juice*
>*¼ teaspoon ground nutmeg*
>*Pinch of ground allspice*
>*Pinch of ground cloves*
>*1¾ cups liquid egg*
>*½ cup skim milk*
>*½ cup old-fashioned rolled oats*
>*¼ cup whole-wheat flour*
>*¼ teaspoon salt*

1. Cut each apple into 8 slices.

2. Heat the margarine in a nonstick skillet over medium heat. Add the apple slices, apple juice, nutmeg, allspice, and cloves. Cook until tender-crisp, about 15 minutes. Place the apple slices in an 8-inch square baking dish and set aside.

3. Preheat the oven to 350°F.

4. Whisk together the liquid egg, milk, oats, flour, and salt in a large bowl. Pour over the apples and bake until the pancake is puffed and golden brown and a knife inserted in the center comes out clean, about 20 minutes.

Speedy Options:
Substitute a large can of sliced peaches or pears in water, drained, for the apples—no cooking required.

Florentine Frittata ●

2 servings

A frittata is an easy Italian omelet that doesn't require flipping. You just pop it under the broiler to finish it off. It also makes a delicious lunch served on a slice of stone-ground whole-wheat toast alongside a tossed salad.

> *2 teaspoons extra-virgin olive oil*
> *1 small onion, diced*
> *2 cloves garlic, minced*
> *1 red bell pepper, stemmed, seeded, and chopped*
> *2 tablespoons chopped fresh oregano or 2 teaspoons dried*
> *1 bag (10 ounces) fresh baby spinach*
> *½ teaspoon salt*
> *1¼ cups liquid egg*
> *¼ cup skim milk*
> *Pinch of black pepper*

1. Heat the oil in a large nonstick skillet with an ovenproof handle over medium-high heat. Add the onion, garlic, bell pepper, and oregano. Cook, stirring, until the onion turns golden, about 5 minutes. Add the spinach and half of the salt, cover, and cook until the spinach is wilted, about 2 minutes.

2. Preheat the broiler.

3. Whisk together the liquid egg, milk, the remaining salt, and the back pepper in a small bowl.

4. Pour the mixture into the skillet, stirring gently to combine with the spinach mixture. Cook, stirring gently, for about 2 minutes, lifting the edges to allow uncooked egg to run underneath. Cook until the top is set, about another 3 minutes.

5. Place the skillet under the broiler for about 3 minutes or until the frittata is golden brown and a knife inserted in the center comes out clean.

Canadian Bacon Omelet ●

1 serving

The smoky flavor of bacon makes this omelet a hit. Serve with fresh fruit and yogurt for a hearty breakfast.

> *1 teaspoon canola oil*
> *½ cup liquid egg*
> *1 tablespoon chopped fresh basil or ½ teaspoon dried*
> *1 tablespoon grated Parmesan cheese*
> *Pinch of black pepper*
> *2 slices Canadian bacon or ham, chopped*
> *¼ red or green bell pepper, stemmed, seeded, and chopped*

1. Heat the oil in a small nonstick skillet over medium-high heat. In a bowl, use a fork to stir together the liquid egg, basil, cheese, and bell pepper. Pour into the skillet and cook until almost set, about 5 minutes, lifting the edges of the omelet to allow uncooked egg to run underneath.

2. Spread the bacon and bell pepper over half of the omelet. Using a spatula, fold the other half over the bacon and pepper and cook for 1 minute. Serve immediately.

Filling Options:
Try other fillings for your omelet, such as ½ cup chopped cooked spinach or Swiss chard or asparagus or ¼ cup light-style Swiss or Havarti cheese. Seafood lovers, try ½ cup baby shrimp or crabmeat.

Shrimp and Mushroom Omelet ●

2 servings

This omelet is a hit with my family on weekend mornings. It would also make a special addition to any brunch table.

> *4 teaspoons canola oil*
> *8 ounces small raw shrimp, peeled and deveined*
> *½ small onion, diced*
> *2 cloves garlic, minced*
> *2 cups sliced mushrooms*
> *2 teaspoons chopped fresh thyme leaves or*
>   *½ teaspoon dried*
> *¼ teaspoon salt*
> *Pinch of black pepper*
> *½ red bell pepper, stemmed, seeded, and thinly sliced*
> *1¼ cups liquid egg*
> *⅓ cup chopped fresh flat-leaf parsley*

1. Heat 1 teaspoon of the oil in a large nonstick skillet over medium-high heat. Add the shrimp and cook until pink, about 4 minutes. Remove the shrimp to a bowl and keep warm.

2. Return the skillet to medium-high heat and add 1 teaspoon of the oil. Cook the onion and garlic for about 2 minutes, or until starting to brown. Add the mushrooms, thyme, salt, and black pepper. Cook, stirring, until all liquid is evaporated and the mushrooms are golden, about 8 minutes. Stir in the bell pepper and add the mixture to the cooked shrimp.

3. In the same skillet, heat the remaining oil over medium heat. In a bowl, use a fork to stir together the liquid egg and parsley. Pour into the skillet and cook until set, lifting the edges to allow uncooked egg to run underneath, about 5 minutes.

4. Spread the shrimp and mushroom mixture over half of the omelet. Using a spatula, fold the other half over the shrimp and mushrooms and cook for 1 minute. Cut in half and serve immediately.

"As a teenager, I know that dieting is a big thing for us. So many of my friends are always trying different diets to lose weight and usually end up going hungry. Because I've seen this so many times, the idea of dieting completely turned me off—until I found your diet. I've been so amazed with the results, I don't want to give away my secret to my friends! I've managed to lose 24 pounds in a healthy, natural way—even my doctor is pleased with what I have done."

—Erika

Southwest Omelet Roll-Up ●

8 servings

B runch is a great time to gather with friends and family, but you don't want to spend all your time at the stove. Here is a family-size omelet with a southwestern-style bean filling that you can make ahead of time. It's perfect with a salad and fresh fruit.

Roux
2 tablespoons canola oil
3 tablespoons whole-wheat flour
1 cup warm skim milk
¼ teaspoon salt
Pinch of black pepper
Pinch of ground cumin (optional)

Omelet
4 egg whites (see Hint)
1 cup liquid egg

Filling
1 package (8 ounces) light cream cheese, softened
½ cup low-fat salsa
1 can (19 ounces) kidney beans or black beans,
*   drained and rinsed*
1 red or green bell pepper, stemmed, seeded, and diced
2 scallions, chopped
¼ cup chopped fresh cilantro or flat-leaf parsley

1. *Make the roux:* Heat the oil in a small saucepan over medium heat and add the flour. Cook for 1 minute, whisking constantly. Slowly add the milk and cook, whisking gently, until thick enough to coat the back of a spoon, about 5 minutes. Whisk in the salt, pepper, and cumin, if using, and whisk to combine thoroughly. Pour into a large bowl and let cool.

2. Preheat the oven to 350°F. Grease an 11 × 17-inch baking sheet and line it with parchment paper.

3. Meanwhile, in another bowl, beat the egg whites to stiff peaks. Whisk the liquid egg into the roux and fold half of the egg whites into the mixture. Add the remaining egg whites, folding gently until combined. Pour the mixture onto the prepared baking sheet. Bake until the eggs are puffed, lightly golden, and firm to the touch, about 18 minutes. Let cool on the baking sheet.

4. *Make the filling:* Combine the cream cheese and salsa in a large bowl and stir until smooth. Stir in the beans, bell pepper, scallions, and cilantro and set aside.

5. Run a small knife around the edges of the baking sheet and place a clean tea towel over the top. Invert the eggs onto a work surface and gently peel off the parchment paper. Spread the filling evenly over the eggs, leaving a 2-inch border on one of the long sides.

6. Using the tea towel as a guide, roll up the omelet, starting with the other long side and working toward the long side with the 2-inch border. Cut in half to make 2 rolls. Using a long spatula or palette knife, transfer the rolls to a large serving platter. Cut each roll into 4 pieces before serving.

Storage:
Cover with plastic wrap and refrigerate for up to 4 hours. Uncover and reheat in a low oven for 20 minutes.

Helpful Hint:
You can use ½ cup liquid egg whites instead of the 4 egg whites.

Green Eggs and Ham ●

6 servings

A beloved childhood story comes to life, with very healthy results. Spinach adds color and flavor to the egg mixture and lean ham adds a salty zing. This is a recipe that begs to be shared with family and friends at a festive breakfast or lunch.

> 1 teaspoon canola oil
> 1 small onion, finely diced
> 1 clove garlic, minced
> 2 red bell peppers, stemmed, seeded, and thinly sliced
> ¼ cup chopped fresh flat-leaf parsley
> 1 teaspoon chopped fresh basil or marjoram or
>   ¼ teaspoon dried
> 6 slices lean ham or Canadian bacon
> 1 tablespoon Dijon mustard
>
> **Green Eggs**
> 1 bag (10 ounces) fresh baby spinach
> 1 teaspoon canola oil
> 2 cups liquid egg
> ½ teaspoon salt
> ¼ teaspoon black pepper
> 2 tablespoons chopped fresh flat-leaf parsley
> 2 tablespoons chopped fresh basil

1. Heat the oil in a nonstick skillet over medium heat. Add the onion and garlic and cook for 3 minutes. Add the peppers, parsley, and basil and cook until the peppers are tender-crisp, about 3 minutes. Scrape the mixture into a 9 × 13-inch baking dish.

2. Spread each ham slice with some of the mustard and place the slices on top of the pepper mixture in a layer. Set aside.

3. *Make the Green Eggs:* Rinse the spinach in a colander and let drain. Heat a large nonstick skillet over medium-high heat. Add the spinach, in batches if necessary; cover; and cook until bright green and wilted, about 3 minutes. Drain again, let cool somewhat, and squeeze any excess water out. Chop the spinach and set it aside.

4. Preheat the oven to 400°F.

5. Heat the oil in a nonstick skillet over medium heat. Meanwhile, in a large bowl whisk together the liquid egg, salt, and black pepper. Add the chopped spinach and stir to combine.

6. Pour the spinach-egg mixture into the skillet and cook, without stirring, until the mixture begins to set around the edges. Lift one of the edges with a spatula and tilt the pan so the uncooked portion flows underneath. Sprinkle the parsley and basil over the eggs and continue cooking until the eggs are just set.

7. Cut the eggs into six portions and spoon one portion of cooked egg onto each of the the ham slices. Cover the dish with aluminum foil and bake for about 10 minutes to warm through.

Storage:
You can cover and refrigerate this dish up to 1 day before baking. Reheat it in a 350°F oven for about 20 minutes, or until hot.

Huevos Rancheros ●

6 servings

These eggs are a spicy way to start the day and are very filling. They are poached to perfection in the oven, so you can enjoy your guests while brunch cooks away.

> *2 teaspoons canola oil*
> *1 onion, chopped*
> *2 cloves garlic, minced*
> *1 small jalapeño pepper, stemmed, seeded, and minced*
> *1 tablespoon chili powder*
> *1 teaspoon dried oregano*
> *1 teaspoon ground cumin*
> *1 can (14.5 ounces) stewed tomatoes*
> *1 cup vegetable cocktail or tomato juice*
> *1 can (19 ounces) black beans, drained and rinsed*
> *1 can (19 ounces) chickpeas, drained and rinsed*
> *1 green bell pepper, stemmed, seeded, and finely*
>   *chopped*
> *¼ cup chopped fresh cilantro*
> *2 tablespoons chopped fresh flat-leaf parsley*
> *6 eggs*
> *6 small whole-wheat tortillas*

1. Heat the oil over medium heat in a large nonstick skillet and cook the onion, garlic, jalapeño pepper, chili powder, oregano, and cumin until the onion starts to soften, about 3 minutes. Add the tomatoes, vegetable juice, beans, chickpeas, bell pepper, and half each of the cilantro and parsley, and bring to a boil. Reduce the heat and simmer until slightly thickened, about 15 minutes. Pour the mixture into a 9 × 13-inch baking dish.

2. Preheat the oven to 425°F.

3. Break 1 egg into a small bowl and carefully slide it onto the bean mixture. Repeat with the remaining eggs, spacing them out like cookies on a baking sheet. Cover the dish with aluminum foil and bake until the whites of the eggs are set (or longer if desired), about 10 minutes. Sprinkle the remaining cilantro and parsley over the dish and serve with the tortillas.

Option:
For a great vegetarian chili, leave out the eggs and cook the tomato and bean mixture until thickened. Serves 4.

SOUPS

Navy Bean Soup ●

4 servings

This recipe comes from Beth F., who went on the G.I. Diet after hearing about it on a local radio show. She and her husband are both enjoying the new way of eating and like having this thick and nourishing soup for lunch.

> *2 cups dried navy beans*
> *12 cups (3 quarts) water*
> *2 carrots, chopped*
> *1 large onion, chopped*
> *1 stalk celery, chopped*
> *1 bay leaf*
> *1 teaspoon salt*
> *Pinch of black pepper*
> *Pinch of ground cumin (optional)*
> *Tabasco sauce, for serving (optional)*

1. Place the beans and 8 cups of the water in a soup pot and bring to a boil. Reduce the heat and simmer, uncovered, until the beans are almost tender, about 1 hour. Add the remaining 4 cups of water, the carrots, onion, celery, and bay leaf and cook until the vegetables and beans are tender, about 1 hour more.

2. Remove the bay leaf. Add the salt and pepper and cumin, if you like. Serve with Tabasco, if desired.

Miso Soup ●

4 servings

This is a great starter for an Asian-inspired dinner. Miso is fermented soybean paste that ranges in color from white to dark brown. The lighter the color, the milder the flavor. Miso tends to sink to the bottom, so to get its full, rich flavor, be sure to stir your soup as you eat it.

4 cups vegetable broth (low-fat, low-sodium)
2 cups water
1 sheet nori (see Hints)
1 cup diced firm tofu
1 cup sliced mushrooms
3 scallions, chopped
3 tablespoons miso paste (see Hints)
1 tablespoon soy sauce

1. Bring the broth and water to a boil in a soup pot.

2. Meanwhile, tear the nori into small bite-size pieces. Add the nori, tofu, mushrooms, scallions, miso, and soy sauce to the pot. Reduce the heat and simmer until the nori and mushrooms are tender, about 20 minutes.

Helpful Hints:
Nori is the flat, black seaweed used to wrap sushi rolls. Look for nori, also known as toasted seaweed, in the international section of your grocery store or check your local Asian grocery. You can find miso in many grocery stores these days. Otherwise, check your local health food store, Asian grocery, or specialty food shop.

Hearty Onion Soup ●

4 servings

This soup is a cool-weather favorite of mine. If you don't have crocks designed to hold French onion soup, you can ladle the soup into microwave-safe bowls and melt the cheese in the microwave. A splash of Tabasco sauce adds a kick.

> 1 tablespoon canola oil
> 6 onions, thinly sliced
> 2 cloves garlic, minced
> ½ teaspoon salt
> 2 tablespoons whole-wheat flour
> 6 cups beef broth (low-fat, low-sodium)
> ½ cup red wine
> 4 tablespoons dry sherry or cognac
> 1 bay leaf
> ½ teaspoon black pepper
> Tabasco sauce, (optional)
> 4 slices stone-ground whole-wheat toast (see Hint)
> 1 cup shredded low-fat Swiss or Jarlsberg cheese

1. Heat the oil in a soup pot over medium heat. Cook the onions, garlic, and salt, stirring often, until the onions are fragrant and beginning to turn golden, about 5 minutes. Reduce the heat to medium-low and continue cooking, stirring occasionally, until the onions are very golden and very soft, about 20 minutes.

2. Add the flour and stir to coat the onions for 1 minute. Add the broth, wine, sherry, bay leaf, and pepper and bring to a boil. Reduce the heat and simmer, uncovered, for 30 minutes. Remove the bay leaf.

3. Preheat the oven to 400°F.

4. Pour the soup into oven-proof crocks. If desired, add a splash of Tabasco to individual servings. Place a slice of toast in each bowl and sprinkle with cheese. Bake until the cheese is bubbly, about 15 minutes. Broil for the last 30 seconds to brown the cheese.

Lighter Option:
For an even lighter soup, omit the cheese and bread.

Storage:
You can make this soup through step 2 up to 3 days ahead. Let cool to room temperature in the pot, cover, and refrigerate. Reheat before continuing with step 3.

Helpful Hint:
To make your own toasts, place slices of whole-wheat bread on a baking sheet. Bake at 350°F, turning once, until dried, about 20 minutes.

Cream of Spinach Soup ●

4 to 6 servings

M any creamed soups contain, as their names suggest, cream. Some others get a creamy texture from the addition of pureed potatoes. This soup calls for pureed white beans, which add fiber, flavor, and creaminess to it, and which keep it green-light. It's elegant enough for company and it's so good that even people who usually don't like spinach enjoy it.

> *1 teaspoon canola oil*
> *1 onion, chopped*
> *1 stalk celery, chopped*
> *1 carrot, chopped*
> *2 cloves garlic, minced*
> *1 tablespoon chopped fresh thyme or 1 teaspoon dried*
> *2 tomatoes, chopped*
> *5 cups vegetable or chicken broth (low-fat, low-sodium)*
> *1 can (19 ounces) cannellini beans, drained and rinsed*
> *1 bag (10 ounces) baby spinach, trimmed*
> *Pinch of salt*
> *Pinch of black pepper*

1. Heat the oil in a soup pot over medium heat. Add the onion, celery, carrot, garlic, and thyme and cook until the onion has softened, about 5 minutes. Add the tomatoes and cook for 2 minutes. Add the broth and beans and bring to a boil. Reduce the heat and simmer for 10 minutes.

2. Meanwhile, finely shred the spinach, then set it aside.

3. Working in batches, puree the soup in a blender until smooth, then return the soup to the pot. Bring to a gentle boil and add the spinach, salt, and pepper. Cook, stirring, until the spinach is tender, wilted, and bright green, about 5 minutes.

Tuscan White Bean Soup ●

4 servings

I first tried this country-style soup in Tuscany and immediately fell in love with it. I serve it in deep Italian ceramic soup bowls and dream I'm back in the Italian countryside.

1 tablespoon extra-virgin olive oil
1 onion, chopped
4 cloves garlic, minced
1 carrot, chopped
1 stalk celery, chopped
4 fresh sage leaves or ½ teaspoon dried
*6 cups vegetable or chicken broth (low-fat,
    low-sodium)*
*2 cans (19 ounces each) cannellini beans,
    drained and rinsed*
4 cups shredded kale
Pinch of salt
Pinch of black pepper

1. Heat the oil in a soup pot over medium heat. Add the onion, garlic, carrot, celery, and sage and cook until softened, about 5 minutes.

2. Add the broth, beans, kale, salt, and pepper and cook, stirring occasionally, until the kale is tender, about 20 minutes.

Cauliflower and Chickpea Soup ●

6 to 8 servings

This combination will help you find another reason to buy cauliflower again—it's absolutely delicious with a hint of ginger and cumin! By pureeing the soup you end up with a smooth, creamy texture that is irresistible.

1 teaspoon canola oil
1 onion, chopped
2 cloves garlic, minced
1 carrot, chopped
1 stalk celery, chopped
1 tablespoon peeled and minced fresh ginger
2 teaspoons ground cumin
½ teaspoon ground coriander
¼ teaspoon ground turmeric
6 cups chopped cauliflower (see Hint)
2 cans (19 ounces each) chickpeas,
    drained and rinsed
6 cups vegetable or chicken broth
    (low-fat, low-sodium)
½ cup nonfat plain yogurt
3 tablespoons chopped fresh cilantro

1. Heat the oil in a soup pot over medium heat. Add the onion, garlic, carrot, celery, ginger, cumin, coriander, and turmeric and cook until the onion has softened and is becoming fragrant, about 5 minutes. Add the cauliflower and chickpeas and cook, stirring, until coated, about 2 minutes. Add the broth and bring to a boil. Cover, and simmer until the cauliflower is tender, about 20 minutes.

2. Working in batches, transfer the soup in a blender or food processor and puree until smooth. Return the soup to the pot and reheat until steaming.

3. Serve with a dollop of yogurt and a sprinkle of cilantro.

Storage:
Once the soup is completely cool you can store it in airtight containers and freeze for up to 1 month or keep refrigerated for up to 3 days.

Helpful Hint:
You will need to buy 1 small head of cauliflower (about 2 pounds) to get 6 cups of chopped cauliflower.

Minestrone ●

6 servings

This soup is one of my favorites because it contains both pasta and spinach, two ingredients I love. Serve it with a sprinkling of grated Parmesan for extra flavor and a few more red pepper flakes to get your blood pumping.

> 2 teaspoons canola oil
> 3 slices Canadian bacon, chopped
> 1 onion, chopped
> 4 cloves garlic, minced
> 2 carrots, chopped
> 1 stalk celery, chopped
> 1 tablespoon dried oregano
> ½ teaspoon red pepper flakes (or more, to taste)
> ¼ teaspoon salt
> ¼ teaspoon black pepper
> 1 can (28 ounces) crushed plum tomatoes
> 6 cups chicken broth (low-fat, low-sodium)
> 1 bag (10 ounces) baby spinach
> 1 can (19 ounces) kidney beans
> 1 can (19 ounces) chickpeas
> ¾ cup ditalini or tubetti pasta
> ⅓ cup chopped fresh flat-leaf parsley
> 2 tablespoons chopped fresh basil (optional)
> Grated Parmesan cheese to taste (optional)

1. Heat the oil in a soup pot over medium-high heat. Add the Canadian bacon and cook for 2 minutes. Reduce the heat to medium and add the onion, garlic, carrots, celery, oregano, red pepper flakes, salt, and pepper. Cook until the vegetables have softened and the onion is golden, about 10 minutes.

2. Add the tomatoes and broth and bring to a boil. Reduce the heat to a simmer and add the spinach, beans, chickpeas, and pasta. Simmer until the pasta is tender, about 20 minutes. Just before serving, stir in the parsley and the basil, if using. Pass the Parmesan cheese at the table, if desired.

Vegetarian Option:
Omit the Canadian bacon and use vegetable broth instead of chicken broth.

Smoky Black Bean Soup ●

4 servings

Whenever I make this soup, my family always asks for seconds. The wonderful flavor of smoked turkey permeates it. Look for smoked turkey legs in the deli section of your grocery store.

> *1 tablespoon canola oil*
> *1 onion, diced*
> *2 cloves garlic, minced*
> *1 jalapeño pepper, stemmed, seeded, and minced*
> *2 cans (15 ounces each) black beans, drained and rinsed*
> *6 cups chicken broth (low-fat, low-sodium)*
> *1 smoked turkey leg (about 1¼ pounds)*
> *¼ cup tomato paste*
> *2 green bell peppers, stemmed, seeded, and diced*
> *1 tomato, seeded and diced*
> *⅓ cup chopped fresh cilantro*
> *¼ cup light sour cream*

(continued)

1. Heat the oil in a soup pot over medium heat. Cook the onion, garlic, and jalapeño pepper until softened, about 3 minutes. Add the beans, broth, turkey leg, and tomato paste and bring to a boil. Reduce the heat and simmer until the turkey meat begins to fall off the bone, about 1 hour.

2. Remove the meat and bone, and set aside. Working in batches, pour the soup into a blender and puree until smooth. Return the soup to the pot over medium heat. Add the bell peppers and tomato and heat until just barely simmering.

3. Meanwhile, remove the turkey meat from the bone, chop the meat, and add it to the soup. Discard the bone. Serve the soup sprinkled with cilantro and a dollop of sour cream.

Ham Option:
You can substitute smoked ham or ham hock for the turkey leg.

Southwest Chicken and Bean Soup ●

4 servings

This has the flavor of a chicken chili but the consistency of a soup. You can make your own nacho chips to serve alongside by cutting whole-wheat pitas into 8 wedges each and toasting them on a baking sheet in a 400°F oven for 10 minutes.

> *1 teaspoon canola oil*
> *1 onion, finely chopped*
> *2 cloves garlic, minced*

2 teaspoons chili powder
½ teaspoon paprika
½ teaspoon ground cumin
6 cups chicken broth (low-fat, low-sodium)
1 can (14.5 ounces) stewed tomatoes
1 red bell pepper, stemmed, seeded, and diced
1 green bell pepper, stemmed, seeded, and diced
12 ounces boneless chicken, finely chopped
1 can (15 ounces) kidney beans, drained and rinsed
2 tablespoons chopped fresh cilantro
2 tablespoons fresh lime juice

1. Heat the oil in a soup pot over medium heat. Add the onion, garlic, chili powder, paprika, and cumin and cook until the onion has softened, about 5 minutes.

2. Add the broth, tomatoes, and bell peppers and bring to a boil. Reduce the heat to a gentle boil and add the chicken and beans. Cook, stirring, for about 8 minutes, or until the chicken is no longer pink inside. Add the cilantro and lime juice before serving.

Option:
Use boneless turkey or chopped raw shrimp or baby shrimp instead of the chicken.

Ham and Lentil Soup ●

4 servings

L entils are staple in my home. They are quick to cook from scratch and very flavorful. If you want to make this soup even faster to prepare (and only slightly less green-light), use canned lentils (see the instructions below).

> *1 tablespoon canola oil*
> *1 onion, chopped*
> *½ cup diced celery*
> *2 cloves garlic, minced*
> *6 cups chicken broth (low-fat, low-sodium)*
> *1 cup dried green or brown lentils*
> *6 ounces Black Forest ham, diced*
> *1 red bell pepper, stemmed, seeded, and diced*
> *2 tomatoes, seeded and diced*
> *2 tablespoons chopped fresh flat-leaf parsley*

Heat the oil in a soup pot over medium heat. Add the onion, celery, and garlic and cook until softened, about 5 minutes. Add the broth, lentils, ham, and bell pepper and bring to a boil. Reduce the heat and add the tomatoes. Cover and simmer until the lentils are tender, about 30 minutes. Stir in the parsley before serving.

Canned Lentil Option:

Use 2 cans (16 ounces each) green or brown lentils. Drain and rinse well. Add with the broth, and cover and simmer until the vegetables are tender, about 20 minutes.

Mushroom, Barley, and Beef Soup ●

4 to 6 servings

A thick, hearty, stewlike soup will warm up everyone on a cold winter's night. This is real comfort food for the soul and the belly.

>*1 tablespoon canola oil*
>*8 ounces extra-lean ground beef*
>*1 onion, chopped*
>*2 cloves garlic, minced*
>*1 pound mushrooms, sliced (see Note)*
>*1 carrot, chopped*
>*1 stalk celery, chopped*
>*1 tablespoon chopped fresh thyme leaves or*
>   *1 teaspoon dried*
>*2 tablespoons tomato paste*
>*1 tablespoon balsamic vinegar*
>*¼ teaspoon salt*
>*¼ teaspoon black pepper*
>*4 cups beef broth (low-fat, low-sodium)*
>*3 cups water*
>*½ cup barley*
>*1 bay leaf*
>*1 can (15 ounces) black beans, drained and rinsed*

1. Heat the oil in a large, deep pot over medium-high heat. Add the beef and cook, stirring, until no longer pink. Reduce the heat to medium and add the onion and garlic. Cook, stirring, for 5 minutes. Add the mushrooms, carrot, celery, and thyme and cook until all liquid has evaporated from the mushrooms, about 15 minutes.

(continued)

2. Add the tomato paste, vinegar, salt, and pepper and stir to coat the vegetables. Add the broth, water, barley, and bay leaf and bring to a boil. Reduce the heat, cover, and simmer until the barley is tender, about 45 minutes. Add the beans and heat through. Remove the bay leaf before serving.

Chicken Option:
You can use ground chicken or turkey for the beef and use chicken broth instead of beef broth.

Note:
Mushrooms come in all shapes and sizes. The best for this soup are your favorites. I make it with white or brown mushrooms (creminis), shiitakes, oyster mushrooms, and even portobellos.

Cioppino ●

3 servings

This Italian-influenced fish stew can be made with whatever happens to be the fresh catch of the day. Adding shellfish such as crab, clams, or lobster makes it impressive enough for entertaining.

> *1 tablespoon olive oil*
> *1 onion, chopped*
> *4 cloves garlic, minced*
> *1 green bell pepper, stemmed, seeded, and chopped*
> *1 can (28 ounces) diced tomatoes, drained*
> *1 cup fish or chicken broth (low-fat, low-sodium)*
> *½ cup red wine*
> *1 teaspoon dried oregano*
> *2 tablespoons chopped fresh basil or ½ teaspoon dried*
> *½ teaspoon red pepper flakes*
> *½ cup chopped fresh flat-leaf parsley*
> *½ pound mussels in the shell*
> *½ pound cod fillets*
> *½ pound large shrimp, peeled and deveined*

1. Heat the oil in a soup pot over medium heat. Cook the onion, garlic, and bell pepper until softened, about 5 minutes. Add the tomatoes, broth, wine, the oregano, basil, red pepper flakes, and ¼ cup of the parsley and bring to a boil. Reduce the heat and simmer for 15 minutes.

2. Meanwhile, scrub the mussels well and remove the beards, discarding any mussels that do not close when tapped. Add the mussels, cod, and shrimp to the pot. Cover and cook for about 5 minutes, or until the mussels are open and the cod and shrimp are firm. Stir in the remaining ¼ cup of parsley and serve.

Thai Shrimp Soup ●

4 to 6 servings

This soup is very versatile; you can make it with chicken or scallops instead of shrimp. If you can't find lemongrass, use 4 large strips of lemon zest.

> *4 cups chicken or vegetable broth (low-fat, low-sodium)*
> *¼ cup peeled and thinly sliced fresh ginger*
> *2 fresh lemongrass stalks (see Note)*
> *1 clove garlic, minced*
> *1 tablespoon minced hot pepper or ¼ teaspoon red pepper flakes*
> *1 pound large shrimp, peeled and deveined*
> *4 ounces rice vermicelli noodles*
> *2 cups bean sprouts*
> *2 scallions, chopped*
> *2 tablespoons rice vinegar*
> *¼ cup fresh cilantro leaves*

1. Place the broth, ginger, lemongrass, garlic, and hot pepper in a soup pot and bring to a boil. Reduce the heat and simmer for 15 minutes. Add the shrimp, noodles, bean sprouts, and scallions. Cook, stirring, until the shrimp are pink and the noodles tender, about 5 minutes.

2. Remove the lemongrass prior to serving.

3. Serve each bowl of soup with a splash of vinegar and a sprinkle of cilantro.

Note:
Look for lemongrass in the fresh herb section of the produce aisle in the grocery store. Cut the top grassy part off and use the thicker bottom part. Hit the stalk with the back of a knife to release some of the juices before cutting.

SALADS

Green Salad with Vinaigrette ●

1 serving

This good basic salad and vinaigrette can be varied endlessly. Just add more ingredients to serve more people.

Basic Salad
1 ½ cups lettuce (romaine, mesclun, leaf, Boston,
  arugula, watercress, or iceberg)
1 small carrot, shredded
½ bell pepper (red, yellow, or green), stemmed,
  seeded, and chopped
1 plum tomato, cut into wedges
½ cup sliced cucumber
¼ cup sliced red onion (optional)

Vinaigrette
1 tablespoon vinegar (such as white wine, red wine,
  balsamic, rice, or cider) or lemon juice
1 teaspoon extra-virgin olive oil or canola oil
½ teaspoon Dijon mustard
Pinch of salt
Pinch of black pepper
Pinch of shredded fresh herb of choice
  (thyme, oregano, basil, marjoram, or mint)

1. In a large bowl, toss together the lettuce, carrot, bell pepper, tomato, cucumber, and onion.

2. *Make the vinaigrette:* In a small bowl, whisk together the vinegar, oil, mustard, salt, pepper, and herb.

3. Pour the dressing over the greens and toss to coat.

Bacon Spinach Salad with Creamy Buttermilk Dressing ●

4 servings

T he classic combination of bacon and spinach is always a surefire hit. This clever version allows you to have the taste you love in a green-light way by using Canadian bacon instead of red-light regular bacon. If you plan to take this salad with you for lunch, pack the greens and dressing separately.

> *6 slices Canadian bacon*
> *1 bag (10 ounces) fresh baby spinach*
> *1 cup cooked chickpeas*
> *4 radishes, thinly sliced*
> *1 cup bean sprouts*
> *1 red bell pepper, stemmed, seeded, and thinly sliced*
> *⅓ cup thinly sliced red onion*
>
> **Creamy Buttermilk Dressing**
> *¼ cup buttermilk or low-fat sour cream*
> *2 tablespoons light mayonnaise*
> *1 tablespoon cider vinegar*
> *2 teaspoons poppy seeds*
> *1 teaspoon Dijon mustard*
> *½ teaspoon sugar substitute*
> *¼ teaspoon each salt and black pepper*

1. Working in batches, cook the slices of Canadian bacon in a nonstick skillet over medium-high heat until crisp. Let them cool, then coarsely chop them.

2. In a large bowl, toss together the spinach, chickpeas, radishes, bean sprouts, bell pepper, and onion.

3. *Make the Creamy Buttermilk Dressing:* In a small bowl, whisk together the buttermilk, mayonnaise, vinegar, poppy seeds, mustard, sugar substitute, salt, and pepper.

4. Pour the dressing over the salad and toss gently to coat. Sprinkle with the Canadian bacon and toss again.

5. *Make ahead:* You can make the dressing up to 3 days ahead and store it in the refrigerator. You can also prepare the salad greens up to 1 day ahead.

Orange Salad Option:
Omit the bacon. Cut the skin and pith from 2 oranges and discard. Slice the fruit into thin rounds and add to the spinach. Serve with Orange Dressing: Omit the buttermilk and add ¼ cup orange juice.

Creamy Cucumber Salad ●

4 servings

This salad is reminiscent of veggies and dip. Use an English cucumber if available; if not, use a field cucumber and remove the seeds.

> *1 seedless cucumber*
> *2 cups grape tomatoes, halved*
> *⅓ cup low-fat sour cream*
> *⅓ cup low-fat mayonnaise*
> *2 tablespoons chopped fresh dill or 2 teaspoons dried*
> *1 small clove garlic, minced*
> *½ teaspoon grated lemon zest*
> *1 tablespoon fresh lemon juice*
> *½ teaspoon salt*
> *½ teaspoon black pepper*
> *¼ teaspoon celery seeds, crushed*

1. Cut off and discard the ends of the cucumber. Cut it in half lengthwise then cut across into thin slices. Place the slices in a large bowl with the tomatoes and set aside.

2. In a small bowl, whisk together the sour cream, mayonnaise, dill, garlic, lemon zest and juice, salt, pepper, and celery seeds. Pour over the cucumber mixture and stir gently to coat.

Options:
This salad is delicious with bell peppers, carrots, radishes, broccoli, or cauliflower instead of tomatoes.

Tangy Red and Green Coleslaw ●

4 to 6 servings

Replacing the traditional mayonnaise-based dressing with a vinaigrette makes coleslaw low-fat and really tangy! This is a great keeper salad for the refrigerator or to tote along to a potluck.

> *4 cups finely shredded green cabbage*
> *2 cups finely shredded red cabbage*
> *2 carrots, shredded*
> *½ cup thinly sliced celery*
> *¼ cup chopped fresh flat-leaf parsley*
> *½ cup cider vinegar*
> *2 tablespoons canola oil*
> *2 teaspoons sugar substitute*
> *1 teaspoon celery seeds*
> *½ teaspoon salt*
> *Pinch of black pepper*

1. In a large bowl, toss together the green and red cabbage, carrots, celery, and parsley.

2. *Make the dressing:* In a small bowl, whisk together the vinegar, oil, sugar substitute, celery seeds, salt, and pepper.

3. Pour the dressing over the cabbage mixture and toss to coat.

Storage:
Cover and refrigerate for up to 2 days.

Creamy Coleslaw Dressing Option:
Whisk together ¼ cup each plain yogurt and light mayonnaise, 2 tablespoons cider vinegar, 1 tablespoon Dijon mustard, 2 teaspoons sugar substitute, ½ teaspoon celery seeds, and ¼ teaspoon salt.

Zucchini Salad ●

4 to 6 servings

Here's a new way to use up the zucchini that might be overrunning your garden. Serve this crunchy salad as a side dish with Grilled Rosemary Chicken Thighs (page 212).

6 zucchini, trimmed
2 red bell peppers, stemmed, seeded, and chopped
¼ cup chopped fresh flat-leaf parsley
¼ cup chopped fresh basil
3 tablespoons balsamic vinegar
2 tablespoons extra-virgin olive oil
2 cloves garlic, minced
¼ teaspoon salt
¼ teaspoon black pepper
4 ounces sliced prosciutto, fat removed

1. Fill a large pot with water and bring it to a boil. Fill a large bowl with ice water.

2. Cut each zucchini in half lengthwise, then cut the halves across into ½-inch-thick slices. Put the zucchini slices in the pot and cook for 1 minute, or until bright green and tender-crisp. Drain the zucchini, then plunge them into the ice water to stop the cooking process. Drain them again, shaking off excess water, and set aside.

3. In a large bowl, toss together the blanched zucchini, the bell peppers, parsley, and basil. In a small bowl, make the dressing: Whisk together the vinegar, oil, garlic, salt, and pepper.

4. Pouring the dressing over the zucchini mixture and toss gently to coat.

5. Cut the prosciutto into thin strips and sprinkle over the salad.

Storage:
Cover and refrigerate for up to 1 day.

Other Meat Options:
Substitute Black Forest ham, smoked turkey, or cooked chicken for the prosciutto.

Mozzarella and Tomato Stacks ●

4 servings

This salad is a classic from the island of Capri, so it's fitting that it shows off the colors of the Italian flag. If fresh basil is unavailable, chop some flat-leaf parsley and sprinkle it over the tomatoes and cheese.

3 small tomatoes, sliced (16 slices)
16 thin slices low-fat mozzarella cheese
16 fresh basil leaves
2 tablespoons extra-virgin olive oil
2 tablespoons balsamic vinegar
1 clove garlic, minced
¼ teaspoon black pepper

1. Top each tomato slice with a slice of cheese and a basil leaf. Place the stacks on a large platter.

2. In a small bowl, make the dressing: Whisk together the oil, vinegar, garlic, and pepper. Drizzle over the cheese and tomato stacks.

Arugula and Roasted Pepper Pasta Salad ●

4 to 6 servings

Peppery arugula is a perfect match for roasted sweet red peppers. Add some chopped cooked chicken, turkey, or ham and you have an easy, flavorful family lunch.

> *Salt*
> *3 cups whole-wheat fusilli or penne pasta*
> *1 large bunch of arugula, trimmed*
> *1 jar (12 ounces) roasted red peppers, drained*
> *2 jars (6.5 ounces each) artichoke hearts,*
> *   drained and chopped*
> *4 scallions, chopped*
> *2 tomatoes, seeded and chopped*
> *¼ cup white wine vinegar*
> *2 tablespoons extra-virgin olive oil*
> *1 small clove garlic, minced*
> *1 tablespoon chopped fresh thyme or 1 teaspoon dried*
> *2 teaspoons Dijon mustard*
> *¼ teaspoon black pepper*

1. Fill a large pot with water, add salt, and bring to a boil. Cook the pasta until al dente, about 7 minutes. Drain the pasta and rinse under cold water until cool. Transfer it to a large bowl.

2. Tear the arugula into bite-size pieces and add it to the pasta. Slice the peppers into thin strips and add to pasta along with the artichokes, scallions, and tomatoes.

3. In a small bowl, make the dressing: Whisk together the vinegar, oil, garlic, thyme, mustard, ¼ teaspoon salt, and the pepper.

4. Pour the dressing over the salad and toss to coat.

Storage:
Cover and keep in the refrigerator for up to 3 days.

Guacamole Salad

4 servings

I've taken all the wonderful flavors of guacamole and put them into this delicious salad. Serve it as a starter for a Mexican-themed dinner, right before your Chicken Enchiladas (page 220) or Beef Fajitas (page 228). Roll any leftovers in a whole-wheat tortilla or stuff them into a pita for lunch the next day.

> 2 avocados, preferably Hass, peeled, pitted,
>   and chopped
> 1 tomato, seeded and chopped
> ½ yellow bell pepper, stemmed, seeded, and diced
> ⅓ cup diced red onion
> ¼ teaspoon grated lime zest
> 2 tablespoons fresh lime juice
> 1 tablespoon canola oil
> Pinch of salt
> 4 cups shredded romaine lettuce
> 1 scallion, chopped

1. In a large bowl, place the avocado, tomato, bell pepper, onion, lime zest and juice, oil, and salt. Toss gently to combine.

2. Divide the lettuce among 4 dinner plates. Top the lettuce with the avocado mixture and sprinkle with the scallion.

Avocado and Fresh Fruit Salad

4 servings

The avocado is a bit of a surprise in this refreshing salad, but it really does go well with fruit, providing a nice color contrast and a rich, creamy texture.

> *4 cups torn red-leaf lettuce*
> *2 avocados, peeled, pitted, and chopped*
> *2 yellow bell peppers, stemmed, seeded, and chopped*
> *1 mango, peeled, pitted, and chopped*
> *1 papaya, peeled, seeded, and chopped*
> *2 scallions, chopped*
> *½ cup chopped fresh flat-leaf parsley*

> **Dijon Vinaigrette**
> *4 tablespoons canola oil*
> *2 teaspoons grated lime zest*
> *2 tablespoons fresh lime juice*
> *2 tablespoons Dijon mustard*
> *2 small cloves garlic, minced*
> *⅛ teaspoon dried thyme*
> *⅛ teaspoon salt*
> *⅛ teaspoon black pepper*

1. In a large bowl, toss together the lettuce, avocados, bell peppers, mango, papaya, scallions, and parsley.

2. *Make the vinaigrette:* In a small bowl, whisk together the oil, lime zest and juice, mustard, garlic, thyme, salt, and pepper.

3. Pour the vinaigrette over the vegetables and toss to coat.

Mediterranean Bean Salad ●

4 to 6 servings

This recipe is a fresh twist on classic bean salad using sun-dried tomatoes. Take it to the next potluck or pack it away for tomorrow's lunch.

> *Salt*
> *8 ounces green beans, trimmed*
> *¼ cup sun-dried tomatoes*
> *1 can (19 ounces) chickpeas, drained and rinsed*
> *1 can (19 ounces) black beans, drained and rinsed*
> *1 yellow or red bell pepper, stemmed, seeded, and diced*
> *1 cup diced sweet onion*
> *3 tablespoons balsamic vinegar (or substitute lemon juice)*
> *1 tablespoon extra-virgin olive oil*
> *½ teaspoon black pepper*
> *½ cup chopped mixed fresh herbs (such as parsley,*
> *   mint, and basil)*

1. Fill a large pot with water, salt it, and bring it to a boil. Add the beans and cook for 3 minutes. Drain and rinse under cold running water to stop the cooking. Cut the beans into 1-inch pieces, place them in a large bowl, and set aside.

2. Meanwhile, pour ½ cup boiling water over the tomatoes and let soak for 10 minutes. Drain, reserving the soaking liquid. Chop the tomatoes and add them to the beans. Add the chickpeas, black beans, bell pepper, and onion.

3. *Make the dressing:* In a small bowl, whisk together the vinegar, oil, 2 tablespoons of the reserved liquid, ½ teaspoon salt, and the pepper. Pour over the salad and toss to coat. Add the herbs and toss again.

(continued)

Storage:
Cover and refrigerate for up to 2 days.

Bean Options:
Use kidney or pinto beans for the chickpeas and black beans.

Corn Option:
Add 1 12-ounce can of corn, drained, to the salad for extra color and flavor.

Tomato, Zucchini, and Wheat Berry Salad ●

4 servings

I love wheat berries because they have a wonderful nutty flavor and have a very low G.I. rating. Cook up a large batch and put the extra in the freezer for another salad or a great addition to soups.

> *Salt*
> *1 cup wheat berries*
> *1 zucchini, chopped*
> *¼ cup sun-dried tomatoes*
> *2 plum tomatoes, seeded and chopped*
> *¼ cup chopped fresh basil*
> *3 tablespoons balsamic vinegar*
> *2 teaspoons extra-virgin olive oil*
> *1 clove garlic, minced*
> *Pinch of black pepper*

1. Fill a pot with water, salt it, and bring it to a boil. Add the wheat berries and cook, covered, until tender, about 1 hour. Drain the wheat berries, rinse them under cold water until cool, and drain again. Place in a bowl.

2. Meanwhile, fill a small pot with water, salt it, and bring it to a boil. Cook the zucchini until just tender-crisp, about 1 minute. Drain the zucchini, reserving the cooking water, and rinse them under cold water. Drain again and add to the wheat berries. Add the sun-dried tomatoes to the reserved water and let stand until softened, about 10 minutes. Drain the sun-dried tomatoes and chop them fine. Add to the wheat berries along with the plum tomatoes and basil.

3. In a small bowl, whisk together the vinegar, oil, garlic, ¼ teaspoon salt, and the pepper. Pour the dressing over the wheat berry mixture and toss to coat.

Storage:
Cover and refrigerate for up to 3 days.

"I have tried it all: Micro Diet, Cambridge Diet, Grapefruit Diet, Cabbage Soup Diet, Slimming Club, Weight Watchers, and on and on. . . . The best thing about this is I'm not on a diet—I am choosing food I like and trying new combinations that really leave me full and not thinking about food all day."
—Beverley

Lemon Dill Lentil Salad ●

4 servings

I really love the combination of lentils and chickpeas in this salad, but you can use other types of beans as well, such as red or white kidney beans. For another twist, add a sprinkle of feta cheese and a few olives.

1 tablespoon canola oil
1 onion, chopped
1 clove garlic, minced
1½ cups water
⅓ cup dried lentils
Pinch of black pepper
1 can (15 ounces) chickpeas, drained and rinsed
1 green bell pepper, stemmed, seeded, and chopped
1 cup chopped cucumber
1 cup halved grape tomatoes
½ cup chopped fresh flat-leaf parsley
4 lettuce leaves

Lemon Dill Dressing
2 tablespoons canola oil
2 tablespoons chopped fresh dill or
   1 teaspoon dried
½ teaspoon grated lemon zest
1 tablespoon fresh lemon juice
¼ teaspoon salt
¼ teaspoon black pepper

1. Heat the oil in a saucepan over medium heat. Add the onion and garlic and cook until the onion has softened, about 5 minutes. Add the water, lentils, and pepper and bring to a boil. Reduce the heat and simmer for 30 minutes, or until the lentils are tender. Drain any leftover water. Let cool completely.

2. Meanwhile, in a large bowl, combine the chickpeas, bell pepper, cucumber, tomatoes, and parsley. Add the cooled lentils.

3. Place a lettuce leaf on each of 4 plates.

4. *Make the Lemon Dill Dressing:* In a small bowl, whisk together the oil, dill, lemon zest and juice, salt, and pepper. Pour over the salad and gently stir to coat.

5. Serve the salad on the lettuce leaves.

Storage:
Cover and refrigerate for up to 3 days.

Full-Meal Option:
Add some cooked chicken, Black Forest ham, or smoked turkey for a heartier meal.

Tabbouleh Salad ●

4 to 6 servings

You often see this salad in the grocery store deli, but it's very simple to make at home, and the homemade is always tastier. I've added chickpeas for more fiber. Use flat-leaf parsley for best flavor.

1½ cups water
1 cup bulgur
½ teaspoon grated lemon zest
2 tablespoons fresh lemon juice
2 tablespoons extra-virgin olive oil
1 small clove garlic, minced
½ teaspoon salt
½ teaspoon black pepper
¼ teaspoon ground cumin
1 can (19 ounces) chickpeas, drained and rinsed
3 plum tomatoes, seeded and diced
¼ cucumber, diced
1 cup finely chopped fresh flat-leaf parsley
½ cup finely chopped fresh mint
1 tablespoon chopped fresh chives

1. Put the water in a saucepan and bring it to a boil. Add the bulgur. Cover, reduce the heat to low, and cook until the water is absorbed, about 10 minutes. Scrape the bulgur into a large bowl. Let it cool.

2. In a small bowl, whisk together the lemon zest and juice, oil, garlic, salt, pepper, and cumin and pour it over the bulgur. Stir in the chickpeas, tomatoes, cucumber, parsley, mint, and chives until well combined.

Storage:
Cover and refrigerate for up to 3 days.

Mediterranean Rice Salad with Tangy Mustard Herb Dressing ●

4 to 6 servings

Here's a great dinner whose leftovers (if there are any) are just as good the next day for lunch. This version is vegetarian, but meat lovers can feel free to add sliced ham or turkey.

> *1½ cups vegetable or chicken broth*
> *   (low-fat, low-sodium)*
> *¾ cup brown rice*
> *¼ teaspoon salt*
> *2 cups lightly packed baby spinach leaves*
> *2 cups shredded red-leaf lettuce*
> *2 tomatoes, chopped*
> *1 can (19 ounces) chickpeas or navy beans,*
> *   drained and rinsed*
> *1 zucchini, trimmed and diced*
> *1 red bell pepper, stemmed, seeded, and diced*
> *1 cup diced cucumber*
> *2 hard-boiled eggs, peeled and quartered*
>
> **Tangy Mustard Herb Dressing**
> *¼ cup rice vinegar*
> *2 tablespoons chopped fresh basil*
> *2 tablespoons chopped fresh flat-leaf parsley*
> *1 tablespoon extra-virgin olive oil*
> *2 teaspoons Dijon mustard*
> *¼ teaspoon salt*
> *¼ teaspoon black pepper*

(continued)

1. Bring the broth, rice, and salt to a boil in a soup pot. Reduce the heat to low, cover, and cook until the liquid is absorbed, about 35 minutes. Remove from the heat and let stand for about 5 minutes.

2. Fluff the rice with a fork and let cool slightly.

3. Meanwhile, put the spinach, lettuce, tomatoes, chickpeas, zucchini, bell pepper, and cucumber in a large serving bowl. Add the rice and toss to combine. Scatter the egg on top.

4. *Make the Tangy Mustard Herb Dressing:* In a small bowl, whisk together the vinegar, basil, parsley, mint, oil, mustard, salt, and pepper.

5. Pour over the salad and toss gently to coat.

Storage:
Keep this salad, undressed, in an airtight container for up to 1 day in the fridge. Add the dressing just before serving.

Option:
For variety, add other vegetables you might have in the refrigerator, such as broccoli, asparagus, grape tomatoes, or mushrooms.

Niçoise Salad ●

4 to 6 servings

Here's a salad that is a meal in itself. You can enjoy fresh grilled tuna instead of canned when available. Look for firm, bright-colored tuna that has no fishy aroma for the freshest taste. Grill for about 2 minutes per side for a perfect rare tuna steak. The tangy mustard dressing gives the vegetables a real kick of flavor.

> *1 pound green beans, trimmed*
> *2 cups torn red-leaf lettuce*
> *2 cups torn Boston lettuce*
> *4 small new potatoes, cooked*
> *2 cans (6 ounces each) chunk white tuna, drained*
> *2 hard-boiled eggs, quartered*
> *1 can (19 ounces) chickpeas, drained and rinsed*
> *1 cup grape tomatoes*
> *½ small red onion, thinly sliced (optional)*
> *¼ cup small pitted black olives*
>
> **Anchovy Mustard Vinaigrette**
> *1 anchovy fillet, minced, or 1 teaspoon anchovy paste*
> *1 tablespoon Dijon mustard*
> *1 small clove garlic, minced*
> *¼ cup white wine vinegar*
> *2 tablespoons extra-virgin olive oil*
> *¼ teaspoon salt*
> *¼ teaspoon black pepper*
> *Pinch of paprika*
> *2 tablespoons chopped fresh basil or flat-leaf parsley*

1. Bring a saucepan of water to a boil. Add the beans and cook until tender-crisp, about 7 minutes. Drain them, and rinse under cold water until cool. Set aside. *(continued)*

2. Spread the red-leaf and Boston lettuce onto a large platter. Cut the potatoes into quarters and arrange them attractively on the lettuce. Add the cooked beans, the tuna, eggs, chickpeas, tomatoes, onion, and if using, olives.

3. *Make the Anchovy Mustard Vinaigrette:* In a bowl, mash the anchovy fillet with a fork and add the Dijon mustard and garlic. Continue to mash to combine. Whisk in the vinegar, oil, salt, pepper, and paprika. Drizzle the vinaigrette over the salad platter. Sprinkle with the basil before serving.

Salmon Option:
You can use 2 cans (6 ounces each) of salmon, drained, instead of the tuna.

Shrimp Option:
You can use 8 ounces of cooked shrimp instead of the tuna.

Grilled Chicken Salad ●

4 servings

You can use chicken hot off the grill for this salad or grill it ahead of time and serve it cold. If you don't feel like fussing with a grill, see the roasting option that follows the recipe. For a totable lunch, stuff the salad into half of a whole-wheat pita.

> *2 tablespoons soy sauce*
> *2 tablespoons canola oil*
> *2 tablespoons chopped fresh cilantro*
> *1 tablespoon peeled and minced fresh ginger*
> *3 cloves garlic, minced*

¼ teaspoon Asian chili paste
    (or substitute red pepper flakes)
4 boneless, skinless chicken breasts
2 red bell peppers
2 yellow bell peppers
6 cups mesclun greens
3 tablespoons rice vinegar
¼ teaspoon salt

1. Preheat an outdoor grill or a grill pan.

2. In a large bowl, whisk together the soy sauce, 1 tablespoon of the oil, the cilantro, ginger, garlic, and chili paste. Add the chicken breasts and toss to coat well. Cover and refrigerate for at least 30 minutes or up to 1 day.

3. Meanwhile, cut the bell peppers into quarters. Discard the stems and seeds. Place the peppers on the greased grill over medium-high heat. Grill until the skins start to blacken, about 15 minutes. Remove to a plate. Place the chicken breasts on the greased grill over medium-high heat and grill, turning once, until no longer pink inside, 4 to 6 minutes per side. Remove to a plate.

4. Chop the grilled peppers and chicken into bite-size pieces. In a large bowl, toss the chicken and peppers with the greens, the remaining oil, the vinegar, and salt.

Storage:
Refrigerate for up to 1 day.

Roasting Option:
You can roast the peppers and chicken instead of grilling them. Place the peppers on a baking sheet lined with parchment paper and roast in a 425°F oven until the skin of the peppers is blackened, about 15 minutes. Add the chicken breasts and roast until no longer pink inside, about 12 minutes.

Jerk Pork Salad ●

6 servings

Jerk is a traditional Jamaican seasoning used to spice up pork, chicken, and fish. Hot peppers give this some bite, and herbs lend flavor that has a cooling effect. Serve the pork with a salad for a meal perfect for those hot summer nights.

3 scallions, chopped
1 large clove garlic, chopped
½ green bell pepper, stemmed, seeded, and chopped
½ red bell pepper, stemmed, seeded, and chopped
1 small scotch bonnet or jalapeño pepper, stemmed
   and seeded
1 tablespoon chopped fresh thyme leaves or
   1 teaspoon dried
1 teaspoon ground allspice
1 teaspoon ground nutmeg
½ teaspoon black pepper
2 tablespoons fresh lime juice
1 tablespoon canola oil
2 pork tenderloins (12 ounces each; see Hint)

Chili Lime Vinaigrette
2 tablespoons apple cider vinegar
2 teaspoons Dijon mustard
2 teaspoons canola oil
½ teaspoon grated lime zest
1 tablespoon fresh lime juice
½ teaspoon sugar substitute
¼ teaspoon chili powder
Pinch of salt
Pinch of black pepper

6 cups mixed baby greens
1 cup halved grape tomatoes
1 cup chopped cucumber
1 can (15 ounces) chickpeas or cannellini beans,
    drained and rinsed

1. Preheat an outdoor grill or a grill pan.

2. In a food processor, combine the scallions, garlic, bell peppers, scotch bonnet pepper, thyme, allspice, nutmeg, and black pepper. Pulse until a smooth paste forms. Pulse in the lime juice and oil.

3. Place the tenderloins in a shallow dish and spread with the jerk seasoning, turning to coat. Cover and refrigerate for at least 20 minutes and up to 8 hours.

4. *Make the Chili Lime Vinaigrette:* In a small bowl, whisk together the vinegar, mustard, oil, lime zest and juice, sugar substitute, chili powder, salt, and black pepper.

5. Place the tenderloins on the greased grill over medium-high heat. Cook, turning occasionally, for about 20 minutes, or until only a hint of pink remains. Remove to a plate.

6. In a serving bowl, toss together the greens, tomatoes, cucumber, and chickpeas. Pour the vinaigrette over the salad and toss to coat.

7. Thinly slice the pork tenderloins and serve on top of the greens.

Storage:
Sliced cooked pork will keep in an airtight container for up to 2 days.

Chicken Option:
Use 3 boneless, skinless chicken breasts instead of the pork tenderloins.

Helpful Hint:
If you only want to cook 1 tenderloin, make the whole amount of the jerk seasoning and only use half. Freeze the rest of the jerk until you want to make the recipe again.

Crab Salad in Tomato Shells ●

4 servings

This makes a great lunch dish. Beefsteak tomatoes are ideal because their large size will accommodate the filling and because their pulp and seeds are easy to scoop out. Try using baby shrimp, tuna, or salmon instead of the crab.

2 cups crabmeat
4 large beefsteak tomatoes
¼ cup light mayonnaise
2 tablespoons light sour cream
½ teaspoon finely grated lemon zest
1 tablespoon fresh lemon juice
2 teaspoons chopped fresh tarragon or
*   ½ teaspoon dried*
Pinch of salt
Pinch of black pepper
1 cup coarsely chopped cooked chickpeas
½ red bell pepper, stemmed, seeded, and diced
¼ cup finely diced celery
¼ cup chopped fresh flat-leaf parsley
2 tablespoons chopped fresh chives
2 tablespoons shredded carrot

1. Place the crabmeat in a fine-mesh sieve and press out any liquid. Remove any cartilage and set the crabmeat aside.

2. Cut the top quarter off of each tomato. Using a small spoon, scoop out the seeds and pulp. Drain the tomatoes cut side down on a plate lined with paper towels.

3. Meanwhile, in a large bowl whisk together the mayonnaise, sour cream, lemon zest and juice, tarragon, salt, and black pepper. Add the chickpeas, bell pepper, celery, parsley, chives, and carrot. Add the crabmeat and stir to combine. Divide the crab mixture among the tomatoes.

Herb Option:

Substitute an additional 3 tablespoons chopped fresh flat-leaf parsley for the chives and tarragon.

Seafood Option:

Substitute baby shrimp, or two 6-ounce cans of tuna or salmon, for the crabmeat.

Crab Melts:

Omit the tomatoes. Top 4 slices of stone-ground whole-wheat bread with the crab mixture and sprinkle with ½ cup of shredded light-style Swiss cheese. Place under the broiler until the cheese is melted.

Shrimp Caesar Salad ●

4 servings

I love Caesar salad as a meal, and by adding grilled chicken breast or roasted salmon fillet you can change the flavor of your meal. Start off with these basic steps to lighten up and make your next Caesar a G.I.-friendly experience. This salad uses garlicky vinaigrette for tons of flavor.

3 slices stone-ground whole-wheat high-fiber bread
2 tablespoons finely chopped fresh flat-leaf parsley
2 cloves garlic, minced
2 teaspoons extra-virgin olive oil
½ teaspoon dried basil
Pinch of salt
Pinch of black pepper
4 cups chopped romaine lettuce
1 can (19 ounces) chickpeas, drained and rinsed
1 cup grape tomatoes, halved
12 ounces large cooked shrimp

Anchovy Garlic Dressing
3 cloves garlic, minced
2 anchovy fillets, finely minced (see Hint)
2 teaspoons Dijon mustard
3 tablespoons chicken broth (low fat, low-sodium)
4 teaspoons extra-virgin olive oil
1 tablespoon fresh lemon juice
¼ teaspoon salt
¼ teaspoon black pepper

1. Preheat the oven to 400°F.

2. Cut the bread into ¾-inch pieces and place them in a bowl. Add the parsley, garlic, oil, basil, salt, and pepper and toss to coat well. Spread the bread onto a baking sheet lined with parchment paper and bake until golden and crisp, about 15 minutes. Let cool.

3. In a large serving bowl, combine the lettuce, chickpeas, tomatoes, and shrimp. Set aside.

4. *Make the Anchovy Garlic Dressing:* In a small bowl, use a fork to mash together the garlic, anchovies, and mustard. Whisk in the broth, oil, lemon juice, salt, and pepper.

5. Pour the dressing over the salad and toss to coat. Sprinkle with croutons before serving.

Helpful Hint:
You can use 2 teaspoons of anchovy paste for the anchovy fillets. Look for it in the dairy section of your grocery store.

Steak Salad with
Peppers and Tomatoes ●

2 servings

Thinly slicing the steak for this salad gives the illusion of a lot of meat while keeping each serving size to the recommended 3 to 4 ounces. This recipe serves two, but you can easily double it for four.

> *2 tablespoons extra-virgin olive oil*
> *2 tablespoons red wine vinegar*
> *1 teaspoon Worcestershire sauce*
> *1 tablespoon chopped fresh thyme leaves or*
>   *½ teaspoon dried*
> *½ teaspoon salt*
> *¼ teaspoon black pepper*
> *8 ounces top sirloin grilling steak, 1 inch thick*
> *3 cups torn romaine lettuce or arugula*
> *1 tomato, cut into wedges*
> *½ red bell pepper, stemmed, seeded,*
>   *and thinly sliced*
> *½ green bell pepper, stemmed, seeded,*
>   *and thinly sliced*
> *¼ cucumber, thinly sliced*
> *¼ cup chopped fresh mint or flat-leaf parsley*

1. Preheat an outdoor grill or a grill pan.

2. In a large shallow dish, whisk together 1 tablespoon each of the oil and vinegar, the Worcestershire sauce, thyme, and a pinch each of the salt and black pepper. Place the steak in this marinade and turn it to coat. Cover and refrigerate it for 30 minutes or up to 1 day.

3. Place the steak on the greased grill over medium-high heat and grill for 8 to 10 minutes, turning once, for medium-rare. Continue cooking the steak to desired doneness. Remove to a plate and cover loosely with aluminum foil. Let it sit for 5 minutes.

4. Meanwhile, in a large bowl, toss together the lettuce, tomato, bell peppers, cucumber, and mint. Whisk together the remaining oil, vinegar, salt, and black pepper. Drizzle over the vegetables and toss to coat.

5. Slice the steak into thin strips and add it to the salad. Toss to combine.

Chicken or Salmon Option:
Substitute 2 boneless, skinless chicken breasts or 2 salmon fillets for the steak.

Helpful Hint:
To take this salad to work, pack the beef and salad separately. At lunchtime, combine the two.

Grilled Shrimp Salad ●

3 servings

The crisp, clean flavor of mesclun complements the light spiciness of the shrimp in this salad. You can use arugula or baby spinach in it too. This dish is a good choice for entertaining friends for lunch. It's easy, and you can vary the amount by just adding more shrimp and greens.

6 cups mesclun greens
1 cup sliced mushrooms
½ red bell pepper, stemmed, seeded,
  and thinly sliced
1 tablespoon canola oil
2 teaspoons mild curry paste or powder
2 teaspoons fresh lemon juice
1 teaspoon peeled and grated fresh ginger
Pinch of salt
12 ounces jumbo raw shrimp,
  peeled and deveined

Orange Dressing
1 tablespoon canola oil
½ teaspoon grated orange zest
1 tablespoon fresh orange juice
1 tablespoon fresh lemon juice
1 teaspoon Dijon mustard
1 tablespoon chopped fresh mint or ½ teaspoon dried
1 small clove garlic, minced
¼ teaspoon salt

1. In a large bowl, toss together the greens, mushrooms, and bell pepper. Set aside.

2. In a shallow dish, stir together the oil, curry paste, lemon juice, ginger, and salt. Add the shrimp and, using your hands, toss to coat the shrimp evenly.

3. Preheat the grill or broiler and lightly oil the grill rack or a baking sheet. If you plan to grill the shrimp, thread them onto skewers (see Hint); if you plan to broil them, spread them on the baking sheet. Grill or broil the shrimp over high heat, turning once, until pink and firm, about 4 minutes.

4. *Make the Orange Dressing:* In a small bowl, whisk together the oil, orange zest, orange and lemon juices, mustard, mint, garlic, and salt. Pour the dressing over the greens and toss to coat.

5. Spread the cooked shrimp over the greens and serve immediately.

Helpful Hint:
Soak wooden skewers in water for 30 minutes before using. This will prevent them from burning before the food is cooked.

Asian Grilled Tofu Salad ●

4 servings

Marinating and grilling the tofu adds lots of flavor to this salad. Have it with a bowl of Miso Soup (page 117) for a terrific lunch.

1 package (14 ounces) extra-firm tofu
¼ cup rice vinegar
3 tablespoons soy sauce
2 tablespoons chopped fresh cilantro
1 tablespoon peeled and minced fresh ginger or
    ½ teaspoon ground ginger
1 clove garlic, minced
¼ teaspoon Asian chili paste or hot sauce
6 cups mesclun greens
1 cup grape tomatoes
½ cup bean sprouts
2 scallions, chopped
2 teaspoons canola oil

1. Cut the tofu in half lengthwise. Repeat with each piece to get 4 long slabs of tofu. Set aside.

2. In a shallow glass dish, whisk together the vinegar, soy sauce, cilantro, ginger, garlic, and chili paste. Add the tofu to this marinade, turning each piece to coat. Cover and let stand for 30 minutes.

3. Preheat the broiler.

4. Meanwhile, in a large bowl, toss together the greens, tomatoes, bean sprouts, and scallions. Set aside.

5. Remove the slices of tofu and reserve the marinade. Broil the tofu slices on a lightly oiled baking sheet, turning once, for about

2 minutes per side, or until golden brown. Watch carefully during broiling to ensure the slices don't burn. Remove to a cutting board and slice into thin strips. Pour ¼ cup of the remaining marinade and oil over the greens and top with grilled tofu.

Storage:
Cover and refrigerate marinated grilled tofu and greens separately for up to 1 day.

MEATLESS

Vegetarian Shepherd's Pie ●

4 servings

Here is a lighter twist on what is usually a quite heavy dish. While a traditional shepherd's pie is filled with ground beef or lamb, ours is filled instead with bulgur and beans. It's still comforting and filled with protein, just healthier. Bulgur is also sold as "Middle Eastern pasta" or cracked wheat. If you like you can skip the potato topping and serve the pie filling in bowls like a chili.

1 teaspoon canola oil
1 small onion, finely chopped
2 cloves garlic, minced
¾ cup bulgur
1 teaspoon dried oregano
½ teaspoon dried basil
1½ cups vegetable broth (low-fat, low-sodium)
1 cup canned stewed tomatoes with juices
2 red new potatoes
¼ cup water
1 can (19 ounces) chickpeas, drained and rinsed
1 cup frozen peas
½ teaspoon salt
½ teaspoon black pepper
2 tablespoons chopped fresh flat-leaf parsley

1. Heat the oil in a nonstick skillet over medium heat. Add the onion, garlic, bulgur, oregano, and basil and cook until the onion is softened, about 5 minutes. Add the broth and tomatoes, breaking up the tomatoes with the back of a spoon, and bring to a boil. Reduce the heat to a simmer, cover, and cook until the bulgur is just tender, about 10 minutes.

2. Preheat the oven to 400°F.

3. Meanwhile, pierce the potatoes all over with a fork. Place the potatoes in a small bowl with the water and microwave on high for 5 minutes. Let cool.

4. Add the chickpeas, peas, and half each of the salt and pepper to the bulgur mixture and stir to combine. Scrape into an 8-inch casserole dish, smoothing the top.

5. Thinly slice the potatoes and layer them, overlapping slightly, on top of the bulgur mixture. Sprinkle with the remaining salt and pepper and the parsley.

6. Bake until the mixture is bubbly, about 20 minutes. Let cool slightly before serving.

Option:
Use veggie ground round instead of the bulgur and reduce the broth to 1 cup.

Boiling Potato Option:
If you prefer not to microwave the potatoes, boil them in a saucepan filled with enough water to cover them for about 10 minutes, or until tender but firm.

Indian Vegetable Curry ●

4 servings

So many wonderful vegetarian dishes come from India. This one has a smooth mild curry flavor, but you can spike up the heat by using a hot curry paste or powder. Serve this with basmati rice.

> *1 tablespoon canola oil*
> *2 onions, cut into wedges*
> *3 cloves garlic, minced*
> *1 tablespoon peeled and chopped fresh ginger*
> *1 tablespoon mild curry paste or powder*
> *1 teaspoon cumin seeds, crushed*
> *3 cups vegetable broth (low-fat, low-sodium)*
> *2 red bell peppers, stemmed, seeded, and chopped*
> *2 cups broccoli florets*
> *8 ounces green beans, trimmed and cut into*
>   *1-inch pieces*
> *1 zucchini, trimmed and chopped*
> *1 can (19 ounces) chickpeas, drained and rinsed*
> *¼ cup chopped fresh cilantro*

Heat the oil in a large saucepan over medium heat. Add the onions, garlic, ginger, curry paste, and cumin seeds and cook until the onions have softened, about 5 minutes. Add the broth and bring to a boil. Add the bell peppers, broccoli, beans, zucchini, and chickpeas. Cover, and simmer for about 15 minutes, or until the vegetables are tender-crisp. Serve hot and top with a sprinkle of cilantro.

Ratatouille ●

4 servings

Ratatouille is a hearty and pleasing vegetable stew from France. I have added beans and tofu to my version of it for protein. If there are any leftovers, add more vegetable broth to make a great chunky soup.

> *1 tablespoon olive oil*
> *1 onion, chopped*
> *4 cloves garlic, minced*
> *½ fennel bulb, trimmed and diced*
> *½ teaspoon dried basil*
> *½ teaspoon dried oregano*
> *1 can (28 ounces) diced tomatoes*
> *2 cups vegetable broth (low-fat, low-sodium)*
> *2 cups diced eggplant*
> *2 zucchini, trimmed and chopped*
> *1 red bell pepper, stemmed, seeded, and chopped*
> *1 can (15 ounces) navy beans*
> *1 can (15 ounces) chickpeas*
> *1 cup diced firm tofu*
> *¼ cup chopped fresh flat-leaf parsley*
> *¼ teaspoon salt*
> *¼ teaspoon black pepper*

1. Heat the oil in a large soup pot over medium-high heat. Add the onion, garlic, fennel, basil, and oregano and cook until the onion softens, about 5 minutes. Add the tomatoes and broth and bring to a boil.

2. Add the eggplant, zucchini, bell pepper, beans, chickpeas, and tofu and return to a boil. Reduce the heat to low and simmer until slightly thickened and the eggplant is very tender, about 30 minutes. Add the parsley, salt, and black pepper just before serving.

Lentil and Rice Filled Peppers ●

4 servings

S tuffed peppers have been around for a long time, and they still make a great meal. You can use any color bell pepper you like.

1 ¼ cups vegetable or chicken broth (low-fat, low-sodium)
¾ cup brown rice
¼ teaspoon salt
¼ teaspoon dried thyme
1 small carrot, shredded
½ zucchini, trimmed and shredded
2 tablespoons chopped fresh flat-leaf parsley
¾ cup low-fat tomato sauce
1 egg
2 tablespoons grated Parmesan cheese
1 ⅓ cups cooked lentils (one 16-ounce can or ½ cup dried)
4 large bell peppers
½ cup water

1. Bring the broth, rice, salt, and thyme to a boil in a soup pot. Reduce the heat to low, cover, and cook for 25 minutes or until the liquid is absorbed.

2. Remove the pot from the heat and sprinkle the shredded carrot and zucchini on top of the rice. Cover, and let the vegetables steam for 5 minutes, or until the carrot is tender-crisp. Scrape the rice mixture into a large bowl, add the parsley, and fluff with a fork.

3. In a small bowl, whisk together ½ cup of the tomato sauce, the egg, and cheese. Pour the mixture over the rice and toss to combine. Add the cooked lentils and toss again. Set the mixture aside.

4. Preheat the oven to 375°F.

5. Cut the top off each bell pepper and remove the seeds and ribs. Trim just enough off the bottom of the peppers to make it flat. Set the peppers in an 8-inch square baking dish and pack each one with the lentil and rice mixture. Spread the remaining tomato sauce on top of the peppers. Pour the water into the dish around the peppers and cover with aluminum foil. Bake for 40 minutes, then remove the foil and return to the oven for another 20 minutes, or until the peppers are tender.

Bean Options:

Try using black beans or pinto beans instead of the lentils. If using canned beans, remember to drain and rinse them before using.

Sweet-and-Sour Tofu ●

4 servings

S weet-and-sour sauce can be sickly sweet if it doesn't have enough sourness or heat to it. This version, however, is well balanced and offers a great blanket of flavor for tofu, which can be rather bland. This dish is also good with chicken or pork instead of tofu.

> *14 ounces extra-firm tofu (see Hint)*
> *1 tablespoon canola oil*
> *¼ cup unsweetened pineapple juice*
> *¼ cup red wine vinegar*
> *¼ cup stemmed, seeded, and minced red bell pepper*
> *3 tablespoons sugar substitute*
> *1 tablespoon soy sauce*
> *1 clove garlic, minced*
> *2 teaspoons peeled and minced fresh ginger*
> *2 teaspoons cornstarch*

(continued)

1. Cut the block of tofu in half horizontally, then cut each half into ½-inch cubes.

2. Heat the oil in a nonstick skillet over medium-high heat. Cook the tofu, turning it several times, until browned on all sides, about 10 minutes. Drain the cooked tofu on a plate lined with paper towels and set it aside.

3. In a saucepan, whisk together the pineapple juice, vinegar, bell pepper, sugar substitute, soy sauce, garlic, ginger, and cornstarch. Cook over medium heat, whisking occasionally, until thickened and bubbly, about 5 minutes. Add the tofu to the sauce and toss to coat.

Helpful Hint:
If extra-firm tofu is unavailable, simply drain firm tofu and place it on a plate lined with a paper towel. Top it with another plate and a heavy can as a weight. Place it in the refrigerator for 4 hours, checking intermittently to drain the liquid. Then proceed with recipe.

Fettuccine Primavera ●

4 servings

Primavera means "spring" in Italian, and you can use your favorite spring vegetables, such as asparagus or peas, in this pasta. Fortunately, you can get peppers, tomatoes, and peas year-round, so you can make this dish anytime.

¼ cup extra-virgin olive oil
2 cups ½-inch cubed firm tofu
Salt
3 cloves garlic, minced
¼ teaspoon red pepper flakes
½ cup vegetable cocktail juice
2 cups chopped fresh asparagus or
 fresh or frozen peas
1 red bell pepper, stemmed, seeded, and thinly sliced
1 carrot, cut into thin strips
1 yellow zucchini, trimmed and thinly sliced
6 ounces whole-wheat fettuccine or linguine pasta
2 plum tomatoes, seeded and chopped
¼ cup chopped fresh flat-leaf parsley
2 tablespoons grated Parmesan cheese

1. Heat 2 tablespoons of the oil in a nonstick skillet over medium-high heat. Cook the tofu on all sides until browned, 5 to 10 minutes. Remove the tofu to a plate and reserve the oil.

2. Bring a large pot of salted water to a boil.

3. Heat the remaining oil and the reserved oil in a large, shallow saucepan over medium heat. Add the garlic and red pepper flakes

(continued)

and cook for 1 minute. Add the vegetable cocktail juice and bring to a boil. Reduce the heat to low and simmer for 1 minute. Add the asparagus, bell pepper, carrot, and zucchini and cook, stirring, until the vegetables are tender-crisp, about 10 minutes.

4. Cook the fettuccine in the large pot of boiling water until al dente, about 8 minutes. Drain the pasta and return it to the pot. Add the vegetables and tofu and toss to coat with the sauce. Stir in the tomatoes, parsley, and cheese just before serving.

Asian Greens and Tofu Stir-Fry ●

4 servings

The wide variety of Asian greens available in grocery stores these days provides excellent new options for old stir-fries. Shanghai bok choy is all green, while the stalks of baby bok choy are white. Serve this with egg or rice noodles.

> 4 scallions
> 2 teaspoons canola oil
> 4 heads baby bok choy, coarsely chopped
> 2 heads Shanghai bok choy, coarsely chopped
> 2 carrots, shredded
> 1 red bell pepper, stemmed, seeded,
>   and thinly sliced
> ¼ cup vegetable broth or water
> 2 tablespoons soy sauce

½ teaspoon toasted sesame oil
19 ounces firm tofu, drained and cubed
1 clove garlic, minced
1 tablespoon peeled and minced fresh ginger
1 tablespoon rice vinegar
1 tablespoon toasted sesame seeds (see Note)

1. Chop the scallions, keeping the white part separate from the green. Heat the oil in a nonstick skillet or wok over medium-high heat. Add the white parts of the scallions and cook for 30 seconds. Add the baby and Shanghai bok choy, carrots, and bell pepper. Stir-fry for another 5 minutes. Add the broth, soy sauce, and sesame oil and bring to a boil. Add the tofu, garlic, and ginger. Reduce the heat to medium, cover, and cook until the vegetables are tender-crisp, about 3 minutes.

2. Drizzle the vegetables with the vinegar and sprinkle with the sesame seeds and reserved scallion.

Note:
To toast raw sesame seeds, heat a dry skillet over medium heat. Add the sesame seeds and, shaking the pan frequently, toast the seeds until they are just starting to darken and pop, about 5 minutes.

Bulgur and Chickpea Chili ●

4 to 6 servings

Bulgur takes the place of meat in this satisfying vegetarian chili. If you cannot find bulgur, which is also known as cracked wheat, in your supermarket, try a health food store or substitute another grain such as brown, basmati, or long-grain rice. (If you do substitute rice, add another 30 minutes to the cooking time.)

1 tablespoon canola oil
1 onion, chopped
4 cloves garlic, minced
2 stalks celery, chopped
1 carrot, chopped
1 tablespoon chili powder
1 tablespoon dried oregano
1 teaspoon ground cumin
2 cans (28 ounces each) diced tomatoes
1 cup vegetable broth (low-fat, low-sodium)
2 cans (19 ounces each) chickpeas, drained and rinsed
¾ cup bulgur
1 red bell pepper, stemmed, seeded, and chopped
¼ teaspoon salt
¼ teaspoon black pepper

1. Heat the oil in a large pot over medium heat. Add the onion, garlic, celery, carrot, chili powder, oregano, and cumin and cook until the onion is softened, about 5 minutes. Add the tomatoes and broth and bring to a boil.

2. Add the chickpeas and bulgur. Reduce the heat to low and simmer until the bulgur is tender, about 20 minutes. Add the bell pepper, salt, and black pepper and cook until thickened, about 10 minutes.

Bean and Onion Pizza ●

4 servings

Here's a restaurant favorite that is custom-made for your G.I. lifestyle. You won't find this thin, crisp pizza at any take-out place. Cooking the onions for a long time over low heat brings out their natural sweetness.

Pizza Dough
¾ cup warm water
2 ¼ teaspoons active dry yeast
1 ⅓ cups whole-wheat flour
½ cup wheat bran
Pinch of salt

Topping
1 teaspoon canola oil
2 onions, thinly sliced
2 cloves garlic, minced
¼ teaspoon dried thyme
Pinch of salt
Pinch of black pepper
¼ cup sun-dried tomatoes
½ cup boiling water
1 cup cooked red kidney beans
¾ cup low-fat tomato sauce
2 tablespoons chopped fresh basil
¾ cup crumbled low-fat feta cheese

1. *Make the Pizza Dough:* Pour the water into a large bowl and sprinkle with the yeast. Let stand for about 10 minutes, or until frothy. Stir in 1¼ cups of the flour, the bran, and salt until a ragged dough forms. Let stand, covered, for 30 minutes. Turn the dough

(continued)

out onto a floured surface and knead it, adding more of the remaining flour as necessary, just until it forms a soft, slightly sticky dough. Place in a greased bowl, cover, and let rest until doubled in bulk, about 1 hour.

2. *Make the Topping:* Heat the oil in a nonstick skillet over medium-high heat. Add the onions and garlic and cook, stirring, until the onions are starting to become golden, about 3 minutes. Reduce the heat to medium and add the thyme, salt, and pepper. Continue cooking, stirring occasionally, until the onions are soft and golden brown, about 15 minutes.

3. Meanwhile, soak the sun-dried tomatoes in the boiling water for 5 minutes. Drain and discard the water and chop the tomatoes.

4. Preheat the oven to 425°F.

5. Punch down the dough and roll it out on a floured surface to fit a 12- to 14-inch round pizza pan. Place the dough on the pan, stretching it as necessary to fit.

6. Put the beans in a large mixing bowl and mash them with a potato masher. Stir in the tomato sauce, sun-dried tomatoes, and basil. Spread the topping over the pizza dough. Top with the onion mixture and sprinkle with the cheese.

7. Bake for about 20 minutes, or until golden and crisp. Cut the pizza into slices and serve.

Make Ahead:
You can make the dough ahead and refrigerate it for up to 12 hours. Let it come to room temperature before rolling it out.

Mushroom and Bean Ragout ●

4 servings

A ragout is a thick sauce that is wonderful served over noodles or rice. I like it served over radiatore or rotini pasta. You can also serve it on its own, enjoying it like a bowl of chili; use it as a substitute for a meat layer in your next lasagna; or use it to fill cannelloni or manicotti shells.

> *2 teaspoons extra-virgin olive oil*
> *1 pound mushrooms, finely chopped*
> *1 onion, chopped*
> *4 cloves garlic, minced*
> *1 small stalk celery, chopped*
> *1 small carrot, diced*
> *1 teaspoon Italian herb seasoning*
> *1 teaspoon paprika*
> *1 can (28 ounces) diced tomatoes*
> *1 can (19 ounces) kidney or cannellini beans,*
> *   drained and rinsed*
> *¼ cup tomato paste*
> *Pinch of salt*
> *Pinch of black pepper*

1. Heat the oil in a large, shallow Dutch oven over medium-high heat. Cook the mushrooms, onion, garlic, celery, carrot, Italian herb seasoning, and paprika until the onion is golden and the liquid from the mushrooms evaporates, about 10 minutes.

2. Add the tomatoes, beans, tomato paste, salt, and pepper and bring to a boil. Reduce the heat and simmer gently for about 25 minutes, or until thickened.

Vegetarian Ground Round Option:
You can use ground meat substitute instead of mushrooms.

Easy-Bake Lasagna ●

8 servings

Though cooking the G.I. way usually means starting from scratch, there are some handy convenience products that are low G.I. Happily, tomato sauce is one of them! This lasagna is great for a crowd. All you need to go with it is a tossed salad.

> *12 whole-wheat lasagna noodles*
> *2 teaspoons canola oil*
> *1 onion, chopped*
> *1 red bell pepper, stemmed, seeded, and chopped*
> *8 ounces mushrooms, sliced*
> *¼ teaspoon salt*
> *¼ teaspoon black pepper*
> *1 bag (10 ounces) baby spinach*
> *1½ cups diced firm tofu*
> *1 cup 1% cottage cheese*
> *⅓ cup liquid egg*
> *1 jar (26 ounces) low-fat tomato sauce*
> *1½ cups shredded part-skim mozzarella cheese*
> *2 tablespoons grated Parmesan cheese*

1. Bring a large pot of salted water to a boil. Cook the lasagna noodles until al dente, about 10 minutes. Drain and rinse under cold water. Lay the noodles flat on damp tea towels and set them aside.

2. Meanwhile, heat the oil in a large nonstick skillet over medium-high heat. Add the onion, bell pepper, mushrooms, salt, and black pepper and cook until the onion is golden brown and the liquid has evaporated, about 8 minutes. Add the spinach and cook, stirring, until wilted, about 2 minutes. Stir in the tofu.

3. In a small bowl, stir together the cottage cheese and liquid egg. Set it aside.

4. Preheat the oven to 350°F.

5. Ladle ½ cup of the tomato sauce in the bottom of a 9 × 13-inch glass baking dish. Lay 3 noodles side by side on top of the sauce. Spread one third of the spinach mixture over the noodles, then do the same with one third of the cottage cheese mixture. Spread with another ½ cup of the tomato sauce and then sprinkle with ⅓ cup of the mozzarella. Repeat these layers twice, ending with noodles on top. Spread the final layer of noodles with the remaining sauce and sprinkle with the remaining mozzarella cheese and the Parmesan cheese. Cover with aluminum foil and bake for 45 minutes. Uncover, and bake for 15 minutes, or until the lasagna is bubbly and a knife inserted into the center is hot to the touch. Let the lasagna cool for 10 minutes before cutting and serving.

Storage:
You can assemble the lasagna and refrigerate it for up to 1 day before baking. You can freeze the baked lasagna whole or in portions and reheat it in the microwave.

Vegetarian Moussaka ●

8 servings

Traditionally made with ground lamb, our moussaka is made low-G.I. by using vegetables. The hearty tomato sauce can be made even more substantial by adding 12 ounces of cooked lean ground beef, lamb, or pork.

2 large eggplants (about 3 pounds total)
2 teaspoons salt
1 teaspoon canola oil
2 large onions, finely chopped
3 cloves garlic, minced
1 red bell pepper, stemmed, seeded, and diced
1 green bell pepper, stemmed, seeded, and diced
1 tablespoon dried oregano
1 teaspoon ground cinnamon
½ teaspoon black pepper
¼ teaspoon ground allspice
1 can (28 ounces) diced tomatoes
¼ cup tomato paste
1 can (19 ounces) chickpeas, drained and rinsed
¼ cup chopped fresh flat-leaf parsley

Cheese Sauce
2 tablespoons canola oil
¼ cup whole-wheat flour
2 cups warm skim milk
¼ teaspoon salt
Pinch of nutmeg
Pinch of black pepper
⅔ cup liquid egg
½ cup 1% pressed cottage cheese
1 cup crumbled low-fat feta cheese

1. Preheat the oven to 425°F.

2. Cut the eggplants into ¼-inch-thick slices and layer them in a colander, sprinkling each layer with some of the salt. Let stand for 30 minutes, then rinse the slices and drain them well. Place them on baking sheets lined with parchment paper and roast, in batches if necessary, for about 20 minutes or until tender. Set aside.

3. Heat the oil in a large, shallow Dutch oven or deep nonstick skillet over medium heat. Add the onions, garlic, bell peppers, oregano, cinnamon, black pepper, and allspice and cook until the onions have softened, about 5 minutes. Add the tomatoes and tomato paste and bring to a boil. Add the chickpeas and parsley, reduce the heat, and simmer for 15 minutes.

4. *Make the Cheese Sauce:* Heat the oil in a saucepan over medium heat. Stir in the flour and cook for 1 minute. Whisk in the milk and cook, whisking gently, for about 10 minutes, or until the mixture is thick enough to coat the back of a spoon. Stir in the salt, nutmeg, and pepper. Let cool slightly and whisk in the liquid egg and cottage cheese.

5. Preheat the oven to 350°F.

6. Spread one third of the tomato sauce in the bottom of a 9 × 13-inch baking dish. Top with one third of the eggplant slices and one quarter of the feta cheese. Repeat the layers. After the last layer of eggplant, spread the cheese sauce evenly over the top and sprinkle with the remaining feta cheese.

7. Bake for about 1 hour or until the top is golden brown. Let stand for 10 minutes before serving.

Tofu Option:
You can use 1 package (12 ounces) extra-firm tofu, diced, for the chickpeas, if desired.

Vegetarian Ground Round Option:
You can add ground meat substitute to the tomato sauce, if desired.

Roasted Vegetable Macaroni and Cheese

4 to 6 servings

Macaroni and cheese is a favorite of all children, so why not add some vegetables for flavor, color, and fiber? Roasting the vegetables brings out their natural sweetness. Look for aged Cheddar that has lots of rich cheese flavor.

2 carrots, coarsely chopped
2 zucchini, trimmed and chopped
2 cloves garlic
1 small eggplant, cubed
1 red bell pepper, stemmed, seeded, and chopped
1 onion, cut into 8 wedges
¼ cup chicken broth (low-fat, low-sodium)
1 teaspoon dried thyme
½ teaspoon salt
¼ teaspoon black pepper

Cheese Sauce
3 tablespoons canola oil
⅓ cup whole-wheat flour
3 cups warm skim milk
2 teaspoons Dijon mustard
1 cup shredded low-fat Cheddar cheese
2 tablespoons grated Parmesan cheese
¼ teaspoon salt
¼ teaspoon black pepper
1½ cups whole-wheat macaroni

1. Preheat the oven to 425°F.

2. In a large bowl, toss together the carrots, zucchini, garlic, eggplant, bell pepper, onion, broth, thyme, salt, and black pepper. Spread the mixture in a single layer on a large baking sheet lined with parchment paper or foil. Roast for about 35 minutes, or until golden brown and tender-crisp. Set aside.

3. Bring a large pot of salted water to a boil.

4. *Make the Cheese Sauce:* Heat the oil in a large saucepan over medium-high heat. Add the flour and cook, stirring, for about 1 minute. Slowly whisk in the milk and continue whisking gently until the mixture is thick enough to coat the back of a spoon, about 5 minutes. Add the mustard, Cheddar and Parmesan cheeses, salt, and pepper and whisk until smooth. Remove from the heat.

5. Meanwhile, cook the macaroni in the boiling water until al dente, about 8 minutes. Drain well and add to the cheese sauce. Add the roasted vegetables and stir to combine.

Storage:
If you want to make this a day ahead, simply put the mixture in a casserole dish, wrap with plastic wrap, and refrigerate. Remove the plastic wrap and bake in a 350°F oven for about 45 minutes or until heated through. (It can also be reheated in the microwave on high in just a few minutes.)

You can also make this ahead in stages. The roasted vegetables will last for up to 2 days in your refrigerator. Allow more time for thorough warming if the vegetables are being added straight from the fridge.

Crusty Top Option:
Pour the macaroni and cheese into a large casserole dish and bake at 350°F until bubbly, about 15 minutes.

Quick-Fix Option:
Substitute 6 cups frozen mixed vegetables, thawed, for the roasted vegetables.

Roasted Pepper and Tomato Strata ●

8 to 10 servings

Stratas, which are casseroles layered with white bread, can be very filling and heavy. Ours calls for a great high-fiber whole-wheat bread, which lends fiber and flavor, and we've cut back the amount to keep things light. A perfect make-ahead brunch idea for a potluck or large gathering.

> *8 slices whole-wheat high-fiber bread*
> *2 jars (12 ounces each) roasted red peppers, drained*
> *4 cups chopped cooked broccoli*
> *1 cup shredded low-fat Swiss cheese*
> *2 cups skim milk*
> *1 cup liquid egg*
> *2 tablespoons Dijon mustard*
> *2 tablespoons chopped fresh flat-leaf parsley*
> *¼ teaspoon salt*
> *¼ teaspoon black pepper*
> *2 tomatoes, sliced*

1. Trim the crusts off the bread. Cut the slices into ¾-inch cubes and sprinkle half in the bottom of a greased 9 × 13-inch baking dish.

2. Slice the peppers into long, thin strips. Sprinkle half of the peppers and half of the broccoli over the bread. Sprinkle with half of the cheese. Top with the remaining bread cubes, peppers, broccoli, and cheese.

3. In a large bowl, whisk together the milk, liquid egg, mustard, parsley, salt, and black pepper. Pour over the bread mixture, cover, and refrigerate for at least 2 hours or up to 24 hours.

4. Preheat the oven to 350°F. Place the tomato slices on top of the casserole, overlapping slightly if necessary. Bake, uncovered, for about 45 minutes, or until the edges are golden and a knife inserted in the center comes out clean.

FISH AND SEAFOOD

Shrimp and Crab Cakes ●

8 to 10 servings

These little cakes are brunch showstoppers. You can use scallops instead of the shrimp and baby spinach for the arugula. However you choose to make them, these will disappear before your eyes.

> 1 can (19 ounces) chickpeas, drained and rinsed
> 1 pound large raw shrimp, peeled and deveined
> 2 cups crabmeat
> ¾ cup fresh whole-wheat bread crumbs
> ⅓ cup liquid egg
> ½ cup finely chopped celery
> ¼ cup chopped fresh dill
> ¼ teaspoon salt
> ¼ teaspoon black pepper
> 2 tomatoes, diced
> 2 red bell peppers, stemmed, seeded, and diced
> 3 tablespoons chopped fresh flat-leaf parsley
>
> **Dressing**
> 1 tablespoon extra-virgin olive oil
> 1 large clove garlic, minced
> ½ jalapeño pepper, stemmed, seeded, and minced
> 3 tablespoons fresh lemon juice
> 4 cups torn arugula or spinach leaves

1. Place the chickpeas in a food processor and pulse until finely chopped. Scrape into a large bowl. Place the shrimp in the food processor and pulse until finely chopped. Add to the chickpeas.

2. Preheat the oven to 425°F.

3. Place the crabmeat in a fine-mesh sieve and press out any liquid. Remove any cartilage and add the crabmeat to the bowl. Add the bread crumbs, liquid egg, celery, dill, salt, and black pepper and use your hands to combine until the mixture sticks together. Form into 18 cakes, each about ½ inch thick. Place the cakes on a baking sheet lined with parchment paper. Bake for about 20 minutes or until golden and firm to the touch.

4. Meanwhile, combine the tomatoes, bell peppers, and parsley in a bowl. Set aside.

5. *Make the Dressing:* In a small bowl, whisk together the oil, garlic, jalapeño pepper, and lemon juice. Set aside.

6. Arrange the arugula on a large serving platter and top with the shrimp and crab cakes. Sprinkle with the tomato mixture and drizzle the dressing over the top just before serving.

Tomato-Topped Shrimp ●

2 servings

T his makes a delicious and attractive dinner for two. Double the recipe to make four servings. Serve this shrimp with rice to sop up all the tomato juices. Brighten up your plate with some asparagus and Mediterranean Bean Salad (page 143). You may replace the shrimp in this recipe with bay scallops if you like.

2 teaspoons extra-virgin olive oil
1 onion, finely chopped
4 cloves garlic, minced
¼ cup chopped fresh basil or flat-leaf parsley
½ teaspoon dried oregano
Pinch of red pepper flakes
¼ cup dry white wine or chicken broth (see Hint)
2 tomatoes, diced
½ cup coarsely chopped cooked chickpeas
¼ teaspoon salt
¼ teaspoon black pepper
8 ounces medium-size raw shrimp, peeled and
    deveined

1. Heat the oil in a nonstick skillet over medium-high heat. Add the onion, garlic, 3 tablespoons of the basil, the oregano, and red pepper flakes and cook until the onion starts to become golden, about 5 minutes. Add the wine and cook for 1 minute more.

2. Add the tomatoes, chickpeas, salt, and pepper. Cook until the mixture starts to thicken, about 8 minutes. Add the shrimp and cook until pink and firm, about 4 minutes. Sprinkle with the remaining basil and serve hot.

Helpful Hint:
The wine in this recipe gives a slightly tangy flavor to the sauce. If you use chicken broth, add ½ teaspoon wine vinegar or cider vinegar to the finished sauce before adding the shrimp.

Sesame Scallop and Black Bean Toss ●

2 servings

Another delicious seafood dinner for two that you can double for four people. Scallops are rich in protein and zinc, but if they are unavailable, you can use jumbo shrimp that have been peeled and deveined.

> 2 tablespoons sesame seeds
> 8 ounces sea scallops
> 2 teaspoons canola oil
> ½ cup thinly sliced red onion
> 1 clove garlic, minced
> 2 cups broccoli florets
> 1 red bell pepper, stemmed, seeded, and sliced
> 1 cup cooked black beans
> 2 tablespoons hoisin sauce
> ¼ cup fresh orange juice
> ½ teaspoon sesame oil
> Pinch of salt
> Pinch of black pepper
> ¼ cup chopped fresh cilantro (optional)

(continued)

1. Place the sesame seeds on a plate. Coat the sides of each scallop with seeds and set aside.

2. Heat the oil in a large nonstick skillet over medium-high heat. Cook the scallops on all sides until just browned. Remove to a plate and cover to keep warm. Leave any remaining sesame seeds in the skillet.

3. Reduce the heat to medium and, in the same skillet, cook the onion and garlic for 3 minutes. Add the broccoli, bell pepper, beans, hoisin sauce, orange juice, sesame oil, salt, and black pepper and cook until the broccoli is tender-crisp, about 8 minutes. Return the scallops to the skillet and heat through. Sprinkle with cilantro, if you like.

Garlic Shrimp Pasta ●

4 servings

G arlic is recognized as being heart healthy. And it is a great decongestant, too. Don't be afraid of the amount of garlic in this dish—the flavor mellows as it cooks.

> *1 tablespoon extra-virgin olive oil*
> *6 cloves garlic, minced*
> *¼ teaspoon red pepper flakes*
> *½ cup dry white wine or chicken broth*
> *(low-fat, low-sodium)*
> *1 pound large raw shrimp, peeled and deveined*
> *½ cup chopped fresh flat-leaf parsley*
> *1 tablespoon nonhydrogenated soft margarine*
> *6 ounces whole-wheat linguine or fettuccine*

1. Bring a large pot of salted water to a boil.

2. Heat the oil in a large nonstick skillet over medium heat. Add the garlic and red pepper flakes and cook just until the garlic starts to turn golden, about 1 minute. Add the wine and bring to a boil. Add the shrimp and cook until the shrimp are pink and firm, about 5 minutes. Add the parsley and margarine and cook until the margarine is melted.

3. Cook the pasta in the boiling salted water until al dente, about 8 minutes. Drain the water and add the pasta to the shrimp mixture. Toss to coat with the sauce.

Quick Fish Steak with Tomato Chickpea Relish ●

4 servings

This recipe is so versatile, you can use fish, chicken, turkey, or my favorite—lamb chops! The slight sweetness of the relish complements the peppery bite of the fish. It's perfect served with basmati rice and green beans.

Tomato Chickpea Relish

2 large tomatoes, seeded and finely chopped
1 cup chopped cooked chickpeas
⅓ cup stemmed, seeded, and finely chopped
  red bell pepper
¼ cup finely chopped onion
¼ cup chopped fresh flat-leaf parsley
¼ cup apple cider vinegar
1 tablespoon sugar substitute
2 teaspoons pickling spice
Pinch of salt
Pinch of black pepper

Fish Steak

¼ cup red wine vinegar
2 tablespoons chopped fresh thyme or 1 teaspoon dried
2 cloves garlic, minced
2 teaspoons Dijon mustard
½ teaspoon black pepper
1 tuna steak (1 pound) or marlin or shark steak

1. Preheat an outdoor grill or a grill pan.

2. *Make the Tomato Chickpea Relish:* In a large bowl, stir together the tomatoes, chickpeas, bell pepper, onion, parsley, vinegar, sugar substitute, pickling spice, salt, and black pepper. Set aside.

3. *Prepare the Fish Steak:* In a large shallow dish, stir together the vinegar, thyme, garlic, mustard, and black pepper. Add the fish steak and turn to coat. Let marinate for 5 minutes.

4. Place the fish steak on the greased grill over medium-high heat and grill for about 8 minutes, turning once, or until medium-rare (or cook to desired doneness).

5. Cut the fish steak into 4 pieces and serve with the relish.

Yellow-Light Option:
Use 8 lean lamb chops in place of the fish steak. Increase the cooking time to 10 minutes for medium-rare.

Green-Light Chicken Option:
Use 4 chicken breasts, skinned, instead of the fish. Increase the cooking time to about 25 minutes.

Almond Haddock Fillets ●

4 servings

A lmonds add calcium to this dish. Serve with Lemon Dill Lentil Salad (page 146), green beans, and rice.

> *½ cup almonds*
> *¼ cup fresh whole-wheat bread crumbs*
> *2 tablespoons chopped fresh tarragon or*
> *   1 teaspoon dried*
> *1 teaspoon grated lemon zest*
> *¼ teaspoon salt*
> *¼ teaspoon black pepper*
> *4 haddock fillets (4 ounces each; see Hint)*
> *1 tablespoon canola oil*
> *Lemon wedges*

1. Place the almonds in a food processor and pulse until they resemble coarse bread crumbs. Remove to a large pie plate or shallow dish. Add the bread crumbs, tarragon, lemon zest, salt, and pepper and stir to combine.

2. Pat the fillets dry using paper towels. Brush about 1 teaspoon of the oil over the fish to coat each fillet completely. Dredge each fillet in the nut mixture to coat both sides.

3. Preheat the oven to 425°F.

4. Heat the remaining oil in a nonstick skillet over medium-high heat. (If you need to, add up to 2 teaspoons of oil so you can coat the skillet for browning.) Cook the fish on both sides just until browned. Place the fillets on a baking sheet lined with parchment paper or aluminum foil and roast for about 10 minutes, or until the fish just flakes with a fork. Serve hot with the lemon wedges.

Helpful Hint:
If you can't find haddock, look for other great white fish such as halibut, cod, tilapia, or whiting. You can also try this mixture on salmon or catfish fillets.

Cornmeal-Crusted Cod ●

4 servings

Cornmeal provides a crunchy, almost nutty texture to fish. Try any of your other favorite white fish in this recipe, such as tilapia or pickerel. Serve with broccoli spears and Tangy Red and Green Coleslaw (page 137).

> *1 cup cornmeal*
> *2 tablespoons chopped fresh dill or 2 teaspoons dried*
> *1 tablespoon grated Parmesan cheese*
> *¼ teaspoon salt*
> *¼ teaspoon black pepper*
> *Pinch of cayenne pepper*
> *4 cod fillets (4 ounces each)*
> *1 egg, lightly beaten*
> *2 tablespoons canola oil*

1. Combine the cornmeal, dill, Parmesan, salt, black pepper, and cayenne in a large, shallow dish or pie plate and set aside.

2. Pat the cod fillets dry using paper towels. Brush each one with egg, then dip into the cornmeal mixture, turning to coat both sides.

3. Heat the oil in a large nonstick skillet over medium-high heat. Add the fish fillets and cook for 3 minutes. Using a spatula, carefully turn the fillets and cook on the other side for another 3 minutes, or until the flesh flakes easily with a fork.

Tuna Patty Melts ●

4 servings

M ake these for lunch at home, or omit the cheese and pack them up for the office. Enjoy with the Creamy Cucumber Salad (page 136) or Lemon Dill Lentil Salad (page 146).

> 2 cans (6 ounces each) chunk white tuna, drained
> 1 dill pickle, finely chopped
> ¼ cup light mayonnaise
> ¼ teaspoon grated lemon zest
> 2 teaspoons fresh lemon juice
> 2 tablespoons finely chopped celery
> 2 tablespoons stemmed, seeded, and diced
>   red bell pepper
> ¼ teaspoon salt
> ¼ teaspoon black pepper
> 2 whole-wheat English muffins
> 4 slices low-fat Cheddar cheese

1. Preheat the broiler.

2. Combine the tuna, pickle, mayonnaise, lemon zest and juice, celery, bell pepper, salt, and black pepper in a bowl.

3. Toast the English muffins in a toaster or under the broiler. Divide the tuna mixture among the muffins and top with the cheese. Place under the broiler for 30 seconds, or until melted.

Bread Option:
You can serve this tuna mixture on 4 slices of stone-ground whole-wheat bread if you like.

Salmon Steaks with Light Dill Tartar Sauce ●

4 servings

The marinade and sauce also go well with other fish, such as halibut, bluefish, or tilapia. Round out the meal with rice and mixed vegetables.

> *1 teaspoon canola oil*
> *1 clove garlic, minced*
> *2 teaspoons grated lemon zest*
> *2 tablespoons fresh lemon juice*
> *1 teaspoon Dijon mustard*
> *½ teaspoon salt*
> *½ teaspoon black pepper*
> *4 salmon steaks (4 ounces each)*

> **Light Dill Tartar Sauce**
> *¼ cup nonfat plain yogurt*
> *¼ cup low-fat mayonnaise*
> *2 tablespoons chopped fresh dill or 2 teaspoons dried*
> *1 tablespoon capers, chopped*
> *1 dill pickle, finely chopped*
> *1 scallion, finely chopped*

1. Preheat an outdoor grill or a grill pan.

2. In a large bowl, whisk together the oil, garlic, lemon zest and juice, mustard, salt, and pepper. Put the salmon steaks in the marinade, turning to coat them well, and let stand for 15 minutes.

(continued)

3. *Make the Light Dill Tartar Sauce:* In another bowl, whisk together the yogurt, mayonnaise, dill, capers, pickle, and scallion. Cover and refrigerate until ready to use.

4. Place the salmon on the greased grill over medium-high heat and grill, turning once, until the fish just flakes with a fork, about 10 minutes. Serve with the tartar sauce.

Grilled Pesto Salmon with Asparagus ●

4 servings

A little bit of store-bought pesto can add a lot of flavor to your food. Here it is combined with mayonnaise to form an intensely flavorful but light crust for salmon. This recipe always gets raves.

> *¼ cup light mayonnaise*
> *2 tablespoons chopped fresh flat-leaf parsley*
> *1 tablespoon pesto*
> *Salt*
> *Black pepper*
> *4 boneless salmon fillets (4 ounces each), skin on*
>   *(see Hint)*
> *1 pound asparagus spears*
> *2 teaspoons extra-virgin olive oil*
> *2 tablespoons fresh lemon juice*

1. Preheat an outdoor grill or a grill pan.

2. Whisk together the mayonnaise, parsley, pesto, and a pinch each of salt and pepper. Spread the mixture evenly over the top of each salmon fillet.

3. Snap the tough ends off of each asparagus spear and discard. Toss the spears with the oil and ¼ teaspoon of pepper.

4. Place the fillets and asparagus on the greased grill over medium-high heat. Close the lid and cook until the fish is firm to the touch and the asparagus is tender-crisp, about 10 minutes. Drizzle the asparagus with lemon juice and sprinkle with ¼ teaspoon of salt.

Fish Options:
This pesto mixture is delicious on halibut, marlin, tuna, or trout.

Helpful Hint:
Leaving the skin on the fillets helps the fish stay moist and keeps it from falling apart.

"I was diagnosed with Type 2 diabetes three years ago. . . . In the year or so since I've been 'Living the G.I. Diet,' my blood sugar levels have gone down to almost normal, my cholesterol levels have improved dramatically, and I'm no longer having to report to the Diabetes Education Center every three months. . . . Thank you for your amazing work."

—Sabine

Ginger Salmon in Parchment ●

4 servings

Cooking in parchment is an easy, healthful way to prepare fish, and the results are moist and flavorful. I find that guests enjoy opening their own packages at the table for a "surprise" dinner.

> *4 cups shredded napa cabbage*
> *1 red bell pepper, stemmed, seeded, and thinly sliced*
> *1 cup snow peas, halved*
> *4 salmon fillets (4 ounces each), skin removed*
> *¼ cup soy sauce*
> *2 scallions, chopped*
> *1 tablespoon peeled and minced fresh ginger*
> *1 clove garlic, minced*
> *1 teaspoon sesame oil*
> *¼ teaspoon black pepper*

1. Cut four large pieces of parchment paper and fold each in half (see Hint). Then unfold them and set aside.

2. Combine the cabbage, bell pepper, and snow peas in a large bowl. Divide the vegetables evenly on one side of the fold of each piece of parchment paper. Place the salmon fillets on top of the vegetables.

3. Preheat the oven to 400°F.

4. In a small bowl, whisk together the soy sauce, scallions, ginger, garlic, sesame oil, and black pepper. Drizzle over the fish and vegetables. Fold the empty half of the parchment over the other half and fold the edges to seal. Place the packages on a large baking sheet and bake until the fish flakes easily, about 20 minutes.

Fish Options:
Try this recipe with any of your favorite fish, such as halibut, tilapia, or snapper.

Helpful Hint:
If you don't have parchment, package these delicious fillets in aluminum foil.

Hoisin-Orange Halibut Steak Packets ●

2 servings

The flavors of hoisin sauce and orange go well together and provide a delicious sauce for delicate halibut. Double the recipe if you are entertaining. You can substitute tilapia, sole, or haddock for the halibut.

4 heads baby bok choy, coarsely chopped
8 ounces shiitake mushrooms, sliced
1 red bell pepper, stemmed, seeded, and sliced
2 cloves garlic, slivered
2 teaspoons canola oil
¼ teaspoon salt
¼ teaspoon black pepper
2 halibut steaks (4 ounces each)
¼ cup hoisin sauce
1 teaspoon grated orange zest
¼ cup fresh orange juice
1 tablespoon chopped fresh flat-leaf parsley

1. Preheat an outdoor grill or a grill pan, or preheat oven to 425°F.

(continued)

2. Combine the bok choy, mushrooms, bell pepper, garlic, oil, salt, and black pepper in a medium-size bowl. Divide the vegetables between 2 pieces of aluminum foil. Top each portion with a halibut steak.

3. In a small bowl, combine the hoisin sauce, orange zest and juice, and parsley. Drizzle this over the halibut steaks. Top with another piece of aluminum foil and seal to form packets. Place the packets on the greased grill over medium-high heat, or in the oven, and cook until the foil packages puff slightly, the fish flakes easily with a fork, and the vegetables are tender, about 20 minutes.

Leek-Stuffed Sole ●

4 servings

Tender leek stuffing gives this fish a burst of flavor. Lemon, olives, and tomato add a touch of the Mediterranean.

> *1 tablespoon extra-virgin olive oil*
> *3 leeks, white and light green parts only, washed, dried, and chopped (see Hint)*
> *3 cloves garlic, minced*
> *1 tablespoon grated lemon zest*
> *1 tablespoon chopped fresh dill or 1 teaspoon dried*
> *¼ teaspoon salt*
> *¼ teaspoon black pepper*
> *4 sole fillets (4 ounces each)*
> *1 tomato, diced*
> *3 tablespoons chopped black olives*
> *2 tablespoons fresh lemon juice*

1. Heat the oil in a nonstick skillet over medium heat. Add the leeks and garlic and cook, stirring occasionally, until softened and golden, about 15 minutes. Remove the skillet from the heat and stir in the lemon zest, dill, and half each of the salt and pepper. Let cool slightly.

2. Place ¼ cup of the leek mixture in the bottom of a small casserole dish. Place the remaining leek mixture in equal portions in the center of each sole fillet; gently fold each fillet over its filling. Lay the stuffed fillets in the dish. Sprinkle the fillets with the remaining salt and pepper.

3. Preheat the oven to 425°F.

4. In a small bowl, combine the tomato, olives, and lemon juice. Sprinkle this mixture over the sole. Bake until the fish just flakes with a fork, about 15 minutes.

Helpful Hint:
To clean the leeks, simply cut the dark green part off and remove any outer layers. Trim the root end. Cut the leek in half lengthwise and rinse under water to remove any dirt. Pat dry and chop.

Pan-Seared White Fish
with Mandarin Salsa ●

4 servings

A quick, bright citrusy salsa lends a tropical note to this hearty fish fillet. You can use tilapia, haddock, or catfish for this elegant meal.

Mandarin Salsa

2 cans (11 ounces each) no-sugar-added mandarin
    oranges, drained
1 red bell pepper, stemmed, seeded, and diced
½ cup diced cucumber
¼ cup finely diced red onion
3 tablespoons chopped fresh cilantro
1 tablespoon rice vinegar
¼ teaspoon salt
Pinch of black pepper

Fish Fillets

¼ cup whole-wheat flour
⅓ cup liquid egg
¾ cup fresh whole-wheat bread crumbs
¼ cup chopped fresh flat-leaf parsley
2 tablespoons wheat bran
2 tablespoons wheat germ
1 tablespoon chopped fresh tarragon or
    1 teaspoon dried
¼ teaspoon salt
¼ teaspoon black pepper
4 white fish fillets (4 ounces each)
4 teaspoons canola oil

1. *Make the Mandarin Salsa:* Coarsely chop the mandarin slices and place them in a bowl. Add the bell pepper, cucumber, onion, cilantro, rice vinegar, salt, and black pepper. Toss to combine.

2. *Prepare the Fish Fillets:* Prepare three large, shallow dishes. In the first place the flour. In the second place the liquid egg. In the third combine the bread crumbs, parsley, wheat bran and germ, tarragon, salt, and black pepper. Dip a fish fillet into the flour first, shaking off the excess. Then coat the fillet with liquid egg. Then dredge it evenly in the bread-crumb mixture. Repeat with the rest of the fillets. Place the prepared fillets on a plate lined with waxed paper and set aside.

3. Heat half of the oil in a large nonstick skillet over medium-high heat. Add 2 of the fillets and cook, turning once, about 10 minutes, or until golden brown. Repeat with the remaining oil and fillets. Serve topped with Mandarin Salsa.

Other Fruit Options:
Try using other fruit such as peaches, nectarines, or mango for a different salsa sensation. You will need 1½ cups of diced fruit.

POULTRY

Cilantro Ginger Turkey Burgers ●

4 servings

You can serve these on whole-wheat bun halves, but they are just as tasty on their own. If ground turkey is unavailable, you can use ground chicken.

> *1 egg, lightly beaten*
> *2 tablespoons soy sauce*
> *2 scallions, chopped*
> *2 cloves garlic, minced*
> *1 tablespoon peeled and minced fresh ginger*
> *⅓ cup chopped fresh cilantro*
> *⅓ cup crushed whole-wheat crackers or*
>   *dry whole-wheat bread crumbs*
> *¼ teaspoon black pepper*
> *1 pound lean ground turkey*

1. In a large bowl, whisk together the egg and soy sauce. Stir in the scallions, garlic, ginger, cilantro, crushed crackers, and pepper. Add the turkey and, using your hands, mix it into the egg mixture until evenly distributed. Shape into 4 patties, each about ½ inch thick.

2. Place the patties in a large nonstick skillet over medium-high heat. Cover and cook, turning once, until no longer pink inside, about 15 minutes.

Turkey and Snow Pea Stir-Fry ●

4 servings

Now that turkey has become more readily available in supermarkets throughout the year, it's not just for the holidays anymore. You can use it instead of chicken in any recipe. In this stir-fry, the turkey takes on a great lemony flavor.

1 pound boneless, skinless turkey breasts
½ teaspoon dried sage
½ teaspoon dried thyme
½ teaspoon salt
¼ teaspoon black pepper
2 teaspoons canola oil
3 scallions, chopped
2 cloves garlic, minced
1 red bell pepper, stemmed, seeded, and chopped
1 cup snow peas, halved
½ cup chicken broth
½ teaspoon grated lemon zest
1 tablespoon fresh lemon juice

1. Cut the turkey into bite-size pieces. Sprinkle with half each of the sage, thyme, salt, and black pepper.

2. Heat the oil in a large nonstick skillet over medium-high heat. Add the turkey and cook until it is no longer pink inside, about 8 minutes. Remove to a plate and keep warm.

3. Return the skillet to the heat and add the scallions, garlic, and bell pepper along with the remaining sage, thyme, salt, and black pepper. Cook until the scallions have softened, about 5 minutes. Add the snow peas, broth, and lemon zest. Bring to a boil, cover, and cook for 1 minute, or until the snow peas are tender-crisp. Return the turkey to the pan and heat through. Drizzle with lemon juice before serving.

Spinach-Stuffed Turkey Breast ●

6 to 8 servings

Veggies are great on the side, but also they add tons of flavor and nutrition when served right in your meat. Try Swiss chard instead of the spinach for a slightly sharper flavor.

> 1 teaspoon canola oil
> ½ cup chopped scallions
> 1 clove garlic, minced
> ½ red bell pepper, stemmed, seeded,
>   and finely diced
> ½ yellow bell pepper, stemmed, seeded,
>   and finely diced
> 1 cup cooked kidney beans, mashed
> 1 tablespoon peeled and finely chopped fresh ginger
> 2 cups shredded spinach
> 2 tablespoons chopped fresh mint
> ¼ teaspoon salt
> ¼ teaspoon black pepper
> 1 boneless turkey breast (about 2 pounds)

Sesame Garlic Marinade

> 3 tablespoons soy sauce
> 2 tablespoons rice vinegar
> 2 cloves garlic, minced
> 2 teaspoons sesame oil
> ½ teaspoon Asian chili paste or Tabasco sauce

1. Heat the oil in a large nonstick skillet over medium heat. Add the scallions and garlic and cook until the scallions are beginning to soften, about 3 minutes. Add the bell peppers, beans, and ginger and cook, stirring, for 2 minutes. Add the spinach, cover, and cook, stirring occasionally, until wilted, about 5 minutes. Remove the skillet from the heat. Add the mint, salt, and black pepper. Let cool completely.

2. Remove the skin from the turkey and discard. Using a chef's knife, slice the turkey breast horizontally in half almost all the way through. Open the meat like a book and, using a meat mallet, pound the turkey to about ½ inch thick. Spread the spinach mixture over the turkey breast. Roll up the meat like a jelly roll, and, using kitchen string, tie the roll at 2-inch intervals. Place the tied roll in a small, shallow roasting pan.

3. *Make the Sesame Garlic Marinade:* In a small bowl, whisk together the soy sauce, rice vinegar, garlic, sesame oil, and Asian chili paste. Pour the marinade over the turkey breast, turning the roll to coat all sides. Cover with plastic wrap and refrigerate for at least 1 hour or for up to 4 hours.

4. Preheat the oven to 325°F. Roast the turkey for about 1 hour and 15 minutes, or until a meat thermometer reaches 180°F. Let stand for 10 minutes before slicing into ½-inch-thick slices. Or let the turkey cool completely and refrigerate until cold. Cut into thin slices and eat cold for lunch.

Grilled Rosemary Chicken Thighs

4 servings

Chicken thighs are cheaper than breasts but are more flavorful and very tender. If it isn't grilling season, bake them in a 400°F oven for about 20 minutes.

> 2 tablespoons extra-virgin olive oil
> 2 cloves garlic, minced
> 2 teaspoons grated lemon zest
> 2 tablespoons fresh lemon juice
> 2 tablespoons dry white wine (see Hint)
> 2 tablespoons chopped fresh rosemary or
>   2 teaspoons dried
> ¼ teaspoon salt
> 8 boneless, skinless chicken thighs

1. Preheat an outdoor grill or a grill pan.

2. In a small bowl, whisk together the oil, garlic, lemon zest and juice, wine, rosemary, and salt. Add the chicken thighs and toss to coat. Cover, refrigerate, and let marinate for 15 to 30 minutes.

3. Place the thighs on the greased grill over medium-high heat. Close the lid and grill, turning once, until the juices run clear when pierced with a knife, about 20 minutes.

Helpful Hint:
You can use 1 tablespoon white wine vinegar or cider vinegar instead of the wine.

Lemon Yogurt Chicken ●

4 servings

This has been adapted from a recipe that Lenna F. sent to us via e-mail. The yogurt marinade keeps the chicken breasts juicy and flavorful. Serve them with Lentil and Rice Filled Peppers (page 170).

1 cup nonfat plain yogurt
1 teaspoon grated lemon zest
1 tablespoon fresh lemon juice
1 clove garlic, minced
Pinch of salt
Pinch of black pepper
4 boneless, skinless chicken breasts

1. In a large shallow dish, whisk together the yogurt, lemon zest and juice, garlic, salt, and pepper. Add the chicken breasts and turn to coat with the yogurt mixture. Cover and refrigerate for at least 1 hour or overnight.

2. Preheat an outdoor grill or a grill pan.

3. Remove the excess yogurt from the chicken and discard. Place the chicken breasts on the greased grill over medium-high heat. Close the lid and grill, turning once, until no longer pink inside, about 12 minutes.

Hunter-Style Chicken

6 servings

Ubiquitously known as chicken cacciatore (*cacciatore* meaning "hunter" in Italian), this dish is a favorite among adults and kids alike. You can use all drumsticks or all thighs if you like.

¼ teaspoon salt
¼ teaspoon black pepper
1 pound skinless chicken drumsticks
1 pound skinless chicken thighs
1 tablespoon extra-virgin olive oil
1 onion, chopped
4 cloves garlic, minced
1 pound mushrooms, quartered
1 red bell pepper, stemmed, seeded, and chopped
1 green bell pepper, stemmed, seeded, and chopped
1 tablespoon dried oregano
1 teaspoon dried basil
¼ cup dry white wine or chicken broth
1 can (28 ounces) diced tomatoes

1. Sprinkle the salt and black pepper over the chicken pieces. Heat half of the oil in a large, shallow pot over medium-high heat. Add the chicken and cook, turning once, until brown on both sides. Remove to a plate.

2. In the same pot, heat the remaining oil over medium-high heat. Add the onion, garlic, mushrooms, bell peppers, oregano, and basil and cook until the vegetables are beginning to brown, about 15 minutes. Pour in the wine and stir the vegetables to deglaze the pan. Add the tomatoes and bring to a boil. Return the chicken to the pot. Reduce the heat and simmer until the chicken is starting to fall off the bone, about 45 minutes.

Thai Chicken Curry ●

4 servings

You can use any color—green, red, or yellow—of Thai curry paste in this hot and spicy dish. If you want it extra hot, increase the curry paste to 1 tablespoon.

> *1 tablespoon canola oil*
> *2 teaspoons Thai curry paste*
> *1 pound boneless, skinless chicken breasts, cut in chunks*
> *1 onion, sliced*
> *1 red bell pepper, stemmed, seeded, and thinly sliced*
> *1 green bell pepper, stemmed, seeded, and thinly sliced*
> *½ cup chicken broth or water*
> *½ cup light coconut milk or light sour cream*
> *2 tablespoons fish or soy sauce*
> *¼ cup chopped fresh basil or cilantro*

Heat the oil in a large skillet or wok over medium-high heat. Add the curry paste and cook for 30 seconds. Add the chicken and stir-fry for 5 minutes. Add the onion and bell peppers and cook, stirring, until the vegetables begin to brown, about 10 minutes. Add the broth, coconut milk, and fish sauce and simmer until the chicken is no longer pink inside, about 10 minutes. Stir in the basil before serving.

Vegetarian Option:
Substitute two 14-ounce packages of extra-firm tofu, cubed, for the chicken, and soy sauce for the fish sauce.

Beef Option:
You can substitute 1 pound of top sirloin grilling steak, thinly sliced, for the chicken, and beef broth for the chicken broth.

Ginger Chicken ●

4 servings

G inger adds a wonderful fresh flavor to this chicken dish. The coriander, cumin, and turmeric give it a beautiful sunny yellow color.

> 2 tablespoons canola oil
> 2 tablespoons peeled and grated fresh ginger
> 1 teaspoon ground coriander
> ½ teaspoon ground cumin
> ½ teaspoon ground turmeric
> ¾ teaspoon salt
> ¼ teaspoon black pepper
> 1½ pounds skinless chicken pieces
> 4 cups cauliflower florets
> 2 carrots, cut into chunks
> 1 red onion, cut into wedges

1. Combine 1 tablespoon of the oil, the ginger, coriander, cumin, turmeric, ¼ teaspoon of the salt, and a pinch of the pepper in a small bowl. Rub the mixture all over the chicken.

2. Preheat the oven to 425°F.

3. In a separate bowl, toss the cauliflower, carrots, and onion with the remaining oil, salt, and pepper. Place the chicken and vegetables on a baking sheet or roasting pan lined with parchment paper. Roast for 35 minutes, or until the juices run clear when the chicken is pierced and the vegetables are tender-crisp and golden.

Chicken Jambalaya ●

4 servings

Jambalaya is a traditional Cajun dish in which rice is used to sop up the rich juices of the stew.

> 2 teaspoons canola oil
> 2 stalks celery, chopped
> 2 cloves garlic, minced
> 1 onion, chopped
> 1 pound boneless, skinless chicken, cut into
>   ½-inch cubes
> 2 teaspoons dried thyme
> 2 teaspoons dried oregano
> 1 teaspoon chili powder
> ¼ teaspoon cayenne pepper (optional)
> 2 cups chicken broth (low-fat, low-sodium)
> 2 green bell peppers, stemmed, seeded, and diced
> 1 can (28 ounces) stewed tomatoes
> 1 can (15 ounces) kidney beans, drained and rinsed
> ¾ cup brown rice
> 1 bay leaf
> ¼ cup chopped fresh flat-leaf parsley

1. Heat the oil in a Dutch oven over medium-high heat. Add the celery, garlic, and onion and cook until the onion has softened, about 5 minutes. Add the chicken, thyme, oregano, chili powder, and the cayenne, if using, and cook, stirring, for 5 minutes.

2. Add the broth, bell peppers, tomatoes, beans, rice, and bay leaf and bring to a boil. Reduce the heat to low, cover, and simmer, stirring occasionally, for about 35 minutes, or until the rice is tender.

(continued)

Let the dish stand for 5 minutes. Remove the bay leaf and discard. Stir in the parsley before serving.

Turkey Option:
Use boneless, skinless turkey instead of the chicken.

Seafood Addition:
Add 8 ounces of small raw shrimp, peeled and deveined, during the last 10 minutes of cooking.

Orange and Chicken Stew ●

4 servings

This dish is based on chicken à l'orange, which was a popular dish for entertaining in the 1970s. It is easy to prepare and has a rich orangey flavor. Serve with rice and a tossed salad.

> *2 teaspoons canola oil*
> *1 pound boneless, skinless chicken breasts,*
> *   cut into bite-size pieces*
> *2 onions, chopped*
> *2 cloves garlic, minced*
> *8 ounces mushrooms, sliced*
> *1 tablespoon chopped fresh rosemary or*
> *   1 teaspoon dried*
> *1 tablespoon chopped fresh thyme leaves or*
> *   1 teaspoon dried*
> *¼ teaspoon salt*

¼ *teaspoon black pepper*
2 *teaspoons grated orange zest*
2 *oranges, peeled and chopped*
1 *cup chicken broth (low-fat, low-sodium)*
1 *bay leaf*
1 *can (19 ounces) pinto beans, drained and rinsed*
1 *green bell pepper, stemmed, seeded, and chopped*
1 *tablespoon cider vinegar*
⅓ *cup chopped fresh flat-leaf parsley*
2 *teaspoons cornstarch*
1 *tablespoon water*

1. Heat the oil in a large, deep nonstick skillet over medium-high heat. Add the chicken and cook, stirring, to brown it. Remove it to a plate. In the same skillet, cook the onions, garlic, mushrooms, rosemary, thyme, salt, and black pepper until the liquid has evaporated, about 8 minutes. Return the chicken to the skillet and add the orange zest, oranges, broth, and bay leaf. Bring to a boil. Cover, and simmer for about 30 minutes, or until the chicken is no longer pink inside.

2. Add the beans, bell pepper, vinegar, and parsley and cook until heated through, about 10 minutes.

3. In a small bowl, whisk together the cornstarch and water. Stir this into the stew and cook until slightly thickened. Remove the bay leaf before serving.

Yellow-Light Pork Option:
You can substitute boneless pork loin for the chicken.

Chicken Enchiladas ●

4 servings

I love having themed dinners, and this recipe is perfect for a Mexican fiesta. Serve these enchiladas with low-fat refried beans and rice for a fun party meal.

2 tablespoons canola oil

2 teaspoons chili powder

1 teaspoon ground cumin

1 teaspoon dried oregano

¼ teaspoon salt

¼ teaspoon black pepper

4 boneless, skinless chicken breasts,
cut into bite-size pieces

2 onions, sliced

1 red bell pepper, stemmed, seeded,
and thinly sliced

1 green bell pepper, stemmed, seeded,
and thinly sliced

1 jalapeño pepper, stemmed, seeded,
and minced

1 cup diced tomatoes

½ cup shredded light-style Cheddar or
Monterey Jack cheese

8 large whole-wheat tortillas

Toppings

½ cup shredded light-style Cheddar or
Monterey Jack cheese

½ cup light sour cream

1. Combine 1 tablespoon of the oil, the chili powder, cumin, oregano, salt, and black pepper in a medium-size bowl. Add the chicken and toss to coat it with the mixture. Heat the remaining oil in a large nonstick skillet over medium-high heat. Add the chicken and cook until no longer pink inside, about 10 minutes. Remove to a plate.

2. Preheat the oven to 400°F.

3. In the same skillet over medium heat, cook the onions, bell peppers, and jalapeño pepper until tender, about 10 minutes. Set aside.

4. Add the chicken, tomatoes, and cheese to the pepper mixture and stir to combine. Divide the filling among the tortillas and roll each of them up. Place them in a shallow 9 × 13-inch greased baking dish. Cover with aluminum foil and bake until the filling is hot, about 15 minutes. Remove the foil and bake for another 5 minutes, or until the tortillas are crisp.

5. Sprinkle with cheese and dollop with sour cream before serving.

Beef Option:
You can substitute 1 pound of top sirloin grilling steak, thinly sliced, for the chicken.

Shrimp Option:
You can substitute 1 pound of large raw shrimp, peeled and deveined, for the chicken.

Basmati Rice Paella ●

6 to 8 servings

This dish is a real crowd pleaser. Have a themed party with other
Spanish foods like wilted greens or stewed chickpeas.

> *1 tablespoon extra-virgin olive oil*
> *1 pound boneless, skinless chicken thighs*
> *1 onion, chopped*
> *4 cloves garlic, minced*
> *1 red bell pepper, stemmed, seeded, and chopped*
> *1 green bell pepper, stemmed, seeded, and chopped*
> *4 cups chicken broth (low-fat, low-sodium)*
> *1 can (28 ounces) diced tomatoes*
> *1 tablespoon paprika*
> *¼ teaspoon saffron threads*
> *1½ cups basmati rice*
> *8 ounces green beans, trimmed*
> *1 cup fresh or frozen lima beans*
> *1 cup fresh or frozen peas*
> *1 pound large raw shrimp, peeled and deveined*
> *1 pound mussels, rinsed (see Hint)*

1. Heat the oil in a large, shallow Dutch oven or a deep nonstick
skillet over medium-high heat. Add the chicken pieces and cook on
both sides until browned. Remove them to a plate.

2. Reduce the heat to medium. Add the onion, garlic, and bell
peppers and cook until the onion has softened, about 5 minutes.
Add the broth, tomatoes, paprika, and saffron and bring to a boil.
Stir in the rice, chicken, and the chicken juices from the plate,
reduce the heat to low, and simmer gently, uncovered, for about 20
minutes.

3. Meanwhile, cut the green beans into 1-inch pieces. Gently stir the greens beans, lima beans, and peas into the rice mixture. Stir in the shrimp and mussels, cover, and cook for about 15 minutes, or until the rice is tender and the mussels are open.

Helpful Hint:
Mussels that do not stay closed before cooking need to be discarded. Simply tap them gently on the counter to see if they will stay closed. Cooked mussels that remain closed must be discarded as well.

Open-Face Chicken Reuben Sandwich ●

4 servings

Hefty reuben sandwiches are a lunch favorite. This version is lightened up, packed with fiber, and spiked with the familiar tangy spread. It's great for lunch or dinner served alongside a hearty salad, followed by fruit for dessert.

Sandwich Spread

½ cup plain yogurt

2 teaspoons balsamic vinegar

1 hard-boiled egg, finely chopped

2 teaspoons minced pitted green olives

2 teaspoons minced red bell pepper

½ teaspoon Worcestershire sauce

4 slices stone-ground whole-wheat high-fiber bread

3 cups shredded cooked chicken (see Hint)

2 cups shredded cabbage

1 tomato, sliced

4 slices low-fat Swiss cheese

2 teaspoons nonhydrogenated soft margarine or
canola oil

1. *Make the Sandwich Spread:* In a small bowl, whisk together the yogurt, vinegar, egg, olives, bell pepper, and Worcestershire sauce.

2. Slather each piece of bread with equal portions of the spread. Top with chicken, cabbage, and tomato. Lay one slice of cheese on each sandwich.

3. Preheat the oven to 400°F.

4. Melt the margarine in a large ovenproof nonstick skillet over medium-high heat. Place the sandwiches in the skillet, in batches if necessary, and cook for about 5 minutes, or until the bread is toasted. Place the skillet in the oven until the cheese melts, about 5 minutes.

Cabbage Option:
If you know you won't use the rest of a whole cabbage after this recipe, pick up a bag of coleslaw mix and use that for the shredded cabbage.

Helpful Hint:
You can use leftover grilled or roasted chicken or turkey. Or you can pick up 2 cooked chicken legs at the grocery store; with skin and bones removed you should have about 3 cups of meat.

MEAT

Beef and Eggplant Chili ●

4 servings

T he addition of eggplant gives this chili a delicious twist. Sprinkle with light-style Monterey Jack cheese for extra zip.

> *12 ounces extra-lean ground beef*
> *1 tablespoon canola oil*
> *2 onions, chopped*
> *4 cloves garlic, minced*
> *2 tablespoons chili powder*
> *1 tablespoon dried oregano*
> *1 teaspoon ground cumin*
> *2 green bell peppers, stemmed, seeded, and chopped*
> *2 cups diced eggplant*
> *1 can (28 ounces) diced tomatoes*
> *½ cup tomato paste*
> *1 can (19 ounces) kidney beans, drained and rinsed*

1. Heat a large saucepan over medium-high heat. Add the beef and cook it, stirring, until browned. Remove it to a plate.

2. In the same saucepan, heat the oil over medium heat and add the onions, garlic, chili powder, oregano, and cumin. Cook, stirring, until softened, about 5 minutes. Add the bell peppers and eggplant and cook until starting to soften, about 10 minutes. Add the tomatoes, tomato paste, and browned beef and bring to a boil. Reduce the heat to low and add the beans. Simmer, covered, for about 1 hour, or until the eggplant is very tender.

Horseradish Burgers ●

4 servings

The combination of beef and horseradish makes these burgers a hit with meat lovers. If you like things spicy, simply smother the top with more horseradish. Serve with a side of Tabbouleh Salad (page 148).

> *1 small onion, grated*
> *1 clove garlic, minced*
> *2 tablespoons horseradish*
> *2 tablespoons steak sauce*
> *1 tablespoon Dijon mustard*
> *1 tablespoon Worcestershire sauce*
> *2 teaspoons dried oregano*
> *½ teaspoon black pepper*
> *¼ teaspoon salt*
> *2 tablespoons wheat bran*
> *2 tablespoons wheat germ*
> *1 pound extra-lean ground beef*
> *2 whole-wheat buns*
> *4 lettuce leaves*
> *1 tomato, stemmed and sliced*
> *¼ cup alfalfa sprouts (optional)*

1. Preheat an outdoor grill, if using.

2. In a large bowl, stir together the onion, garlic, horseradish, steak sauce, mustard, Worcestershire sauce, oregano, pepper, and salt. Add the wheat bran and germ and stir to coat. Let stand for 5 minutes. Using your hands, add the beef and work it into the mixture until well combined.

(continued)

3. Form the meat mixture into 4 patties, each about ½ inch thick. Place them on the greased grill or in a nonstick skillet and cook, turning once, until no longer pink inside, about 12 minutes. Place each patty on one half of a bun. Top with lettuce, tomato slices, and sprouts (if using).

Beef Fajitas ●

2 servings

Here is a restaurant classic that is simple to make at home and simple to double or triple for crowds! Serve the fajitas sizzling from the skillet for great effect.

> *1 teaspoon canola oil*
> *8 ounces top sirloin grilling steak, thinly sliced*
> *1 tablespoon Worcestershire sauce*
> *Pinch of cayenne pepper*
> *1 red onion, sliced*
> *2 cloves garlic, minced*
> *1 red bell pepper, stemmed, seeded, and sliced*
> *1 green bell pepper, stemmed, seeded, and sliced*
> *2 teaspoons chili powder*
> *½ teaspoon ground cumin*
> *½ teaspoon dried thyme*
> *¼ teaspoon salt*
> *¼ teaspoon black pepper*
> *¼ cup low-fat tomato sauce or low-fat salsa*
> *4 small whole-wheat tortillas*
> *¼ cup light sour cream*

1. Heat the oil in a large nonstick skillet over medium-high heat. Add the steak, Worcestershire sauce, and cayenne and cook, turning the slices, until the meat is browned, about 5 minutes. Remove to a plate.

2. Return the skillet to medium heat and add the onion, garlic, bell peppers, chili powder, cumin, thyme, salt, and black pepper. Cook until the peppers are tender-crisp, about 8 minutes. Add the tomato sauce and cook for 5 minutes more. Return the beef to the pan and cook until heated through.

3. Divide the meat mixture among the tortillas, add a dollop of sour cream to each, and roll up.

Poultry Options:
You can use boneless, skinless chicken or turkey breast instead of the beef.

Serving Option:
You can serve the meat mixture over rice instead of filling the tortillas.

Steak Fettuccine ●

4 servings

A steak with a serving of pasta sounds like old-fashioned, heavy fare. Not our version. The meat is marinated with a peppery dressing and served, sliced, atop fettuccine dressed with a fresh tomato sauce. The result is light and flavorful, yet elegant enough for company.

1 top sirloin grilling steak (1 pound)
2 tablespoons Dijon mustard
2 teaspoons dried Italian herb seasoning
½ teaspoon black pepper
1 teaspoon extra-virgin olive oil
2 shallots, thinly sliced
2 cloves garlic, minced
1 teaspoon dried oregano
½ teaspoon dried basil
3 tomatoes, chopped
1 red bell pepper, stemmed, seeded, and thinly sliced
1 orange bell pepper, stemmed, seeded,
    and thinly sliced
½ cup beef broth (low-fat, low-sodium)
1 cup snow peas, trimmed
6 ounces whole-wheat fettuccine or linguine
¼ teaspoon salt

1. Preheat an outdoor grill or a grill pan.

2. Trim any fat from the steak and discard.

3. In a small bowl, stir together the mustard, Italian herb seasoning, and black pepper. Spread evenly over the steak. Place the steak on the greased grill over medium-high heat and grill for about 8 minutes, turning once, or until medium-rare. Remove to a plate, cover, and keep warm.

4. Bring a large pot of salted water to a boil.

5. Heat the oil in a nonstick skillet over medium-high heat. Add the shallots, garlic, oregano, and basil and cook until the shallots are starting to become golden, about 5 minutes. Add the tomatoes, bell peppers and broth and bring to a boil. Reduce the heat and simmer gently until the tomatoes are starting to break down, about 5 minutes. Add the snow peas and cook until bright green, about 3 minutes. Stir in the salt.

6. Cook the fettuccine in the boiling salted water until al dente, about 10 minutes. Drain well and return the pasta to the pot. Toss with the sauce to coat. Place the pasta in a large serving dish. Thinly slice the steak across the grain and lay on top of the fettuccine. Serve immediately.

Pan-Sear Option:
No grill? No problem. Put a little oil in a hot grill pan or cast-iron skillet. Add the steak and cook to desired doneness.

Spaghetti and Meatballs ●

4 servings

A home-cooked meal is a wonderful thing to come home to, and this one is a favorite of many. Make the meatballs ahead and freeze them for a quick after-work meal or an Italian meatball open-face sandwich for lunch.

> *1 egg*
> *⅓ cup fresh whole-wheat bread crumbs*
> *¼ cup wheat bran*
> *¼ cup chopped fresh flat-leaf parsley*
> *1 clove garlic, minced*
> *¼ teaspoon salt*
> *¼ teaspoon black pepper*
> *12 ounces lean ground turkey or chicken*
> *2 cups low-fat chunky vegetable pasta sauce*
> *1 cup cooked chickpeas*
> *½ green bell pepper, stemmed, seeded, and diced*
> *8 ounces whole-wheat spaghetti*

1. Preheat the oven to 350°F.

2. In a large bowl, stir together the egg, bread crumbs, wheat bran, parsley, garlic, salt, and black pepper. Work the ground turkey in with your hands until well combined. Roll the mixture into 1-inch round meatballs and place on a baking sheet lined with aluminum foil. Bake for about 12 minutes, or until no longer pink inside.

3. Meanwhile, bring a large pot of salted water to a boil.

4. In a separate large saucepan, cook the pasta sauce, chickpeas, and bell pepper over medium heat. Add the meatballs and simmer for 15 minutes.

5. Cook the pasta in the boiling water until al dente, about 10 minutes. Remove the meatballs to a small serving bowl. Drain the pasta and add it to the pasta sauce, tossing to coat well. Serve with the meatballs.

Storage:
After baking, let the meatballs cool completely, then freeze in an airtight container for up to 2 months.

Beefy Meatballs ●

About 24 meatballs, enough for 6 servings

You can use ground pork, veal, chicken, or turkey instead of the beef in this recipe. Serve the meatballs on their own or with your favorite low-fat pasta sauce and whole-wheat spaghetti.

> *1 egg*
> *½ cup crushed whole-wheat crackers*
> *⅓ cup chopped fresh flat-leaf parsley*
> *2 tablespoons grated Parmesan cheese*
> *2 tablespoons wheat germ or wheat bran*
> *2 cloves garlic, minced*
> *½ teaspoon salt*
> *¼ teaspoon red pepper flakes*
> *1½ pounds extra-lean ground beef*

1. In a large bowl, whisk the egg with a fork. Add the crushed crackers, parsley, cheese, wheat germ, garlic, salt, and red pepper flakes and stir to combine. Add the meat and combine well, using your hands to distribute the ingredients evenly.

(continued)

2. Preheat the oven to 400°F.

3. Roll the meat mixture into 1-inch balls and place on a baking sheet lined with aluminum foil. Bake for 20 minutes or until the meatballs are no longer pink inside.

Storage:
Let the meatballs cool completely. Place in an airtight container or freezer bag and freeze for up to 2 months.

Mini Meatball Option:
Use a teaspoon measure to make tiny meatballs for your family. These will cook in much less time, about 10 minutes.

Easy Meat Sauce ●

About 5½ cups

This is a great make-ahead recipe. Half of this recipe served over 6 ounces of whole-wheat pasta makes a simple dinner for four. Use the rest in lasagna or even eat it on its own like chili.

> *12 ounces extra-lean ground beef*
> *1 tablespoon canola oil*
> *1 onion, chopped*
> *2 cloves garlic, chopped*
> *1 tablespoon dried oregano*
> *1 teaspoon salt*
> *¼ teaspoon red pepper flakes*
> *2 cans (28 ounces each) plum tomatoes, pureed*
> *1 red bell pepper, stemmed, seeded, and chopped*
> *1 green bell pepper, stemmed, seeded, and chopped*
> *4 fresh basil leaves*
> *4 sprigs fresh flat-leaf parsley*

1. In a deep pot, cook the beef over medium-high heat, stirring constantly, until browned, about 8 minutes. Remove to a plate.

2. In the same pot, reduce the heat to medium and add the oil, onion, garlic, oregano, salt, and red pepper flakes. Cook, stirring, until the onion has softened, about 5 minutes.

3. Add the tomatoes, bell peppers, basil, and parsley and bring to a boil. Return the meat to the sauce. Reduce the heat to low and simmer until thickened, about 30 minutes.

Storage:
Let the mixture cool completely and store in airtight containers. Freeze for up to 1 month.

Spicy Beef and Beans ●

4 servings

This dish is mildly spicy and goes well with pasta and Tangy Red and Green Coleslaw (page 137).

1 tablespoon canola oil
1 pound lean stewing beef, cut into 1-inch cubes
1 onion, chopped
1 carrot, chopped
2 cloves garlic, minced
8 ounces mushrooms, sliced
1 teaspoon dried thyme leaves
½ teaspoon red pepper flakes
2 cups beef broth (low-fat, low-sodium)
¼ cup tomato paste
1 tablespoon Worcestershire sauce
1 bay leaf
1 can (19 ounces) navy beans, drained and rinsed
1 red bell pepper, stemmed, seeded, and chopped
½ teaspoon salt
¼ teaspoon black pepper
¼ cup chopped fresh basil or flat-leaf parsley

1. Heat half of the oil in a large, shallow saucepan over medium-high heat. Add the beef and cook, stirring often, until the pieces are brown on all sides. Remove to a plate and set aside.

2. Return the saucepan to medium heat and add the remaining oil. Add the onion, carrot, garlic, mushrooms, thyme, and red pepper flakes and cook until the onion is golden, about 8 minutes. Add the broth, tomato paste, Worcestershire sauce, bay leaf, and browned beef and their juices and bring to a boil. Reduce the heat, cover, and simmer for 1 hour.

3. Uncover, and add the beans, bell pepper, salt, and black pepper. Cover, and return to a simmer for 1 hour, or until the beef is very tender. Remove the bay leaf and stir in the basil before serving.

Yellow-Light Lamb Option:
You can substitute cubed lamb for the beef.

Lazy Cabbage Rolls ●

6 servings

Making traditional cabbage rolls can be a time-consuming process. If you aren't up to the task but want to enjoy the same great flavor, this is the dish for you. It has all the same ingredients but takes less than half the time to make.

> *2 teaspoons canola oil*
> *1 onion, chopped*
> *2 cloves garlic, minced*
> *¾ cup basmati rice*
> *1½ cups beef or chicken broth (low-fat, low-sodium)*
> *½ teaspoon salt*
> *¼ teaspoon black pepper*
> *12 ounces extra-lean ground beef*
> *½ teaspoon fennel or caraway seeds, crushed*
> *½ teaspoon dried oregano*
> *⅓ cup liquid egg*
> *¼ cup chopped fresh flat-leaf parsley*
> *1 jar (26 ounces) low-fat tomato sauce*
> *6 cups shredded cabbage*
> *½ cup water*

(continued)

1. Heat the oil in a small pot over medium heat. Add the onion and garlic and cook for about 3 minutes, or until softened. Add the rice and stir to combine. Pour in the broth and half each of the salt and pepper and bring to boil. Cover, and reduce the heat to low. Simmer until the liquid is absorbed, about 15 minutes. Scrape the rice into a large bowl and fluff with a fork. Set aside.

2. In a nonstick skillet over medium-high heat, cook the beef, fennel, oregano, and remaining salt and pepper, stirring frequently, just until the beef is browned and cooked through. Add this to the rice mixture along with the liquid egg and parsley and stir until combined.

3. Preheat the oven to 350°F.

4. Spread ½ cup of the tomato sauce in the bottom of a 9 × 13-inch baking dish. Sprinkle one third of the cabbage over the bottom. Spread with half of the rice mixture. Spread with another ½ cup of the tomato sauce. Sprinkle with another third of the cabbage and the remaining rice mixture. Finish with the remaining cabbage, packing down gently. Spread with the remaining tomato sauce and pour the water evenly over the top. Cover with aluminum foil and bake for 1 hour, or until the cabbage is tender.

Poultry Options:
You can substitute ground chicken or turkey for the beef.

Spice Options:
You can use a combination of ¼ teaspoon of crushed anise seeds and ¼ teaspoon of celery seeds, if you don't have fennel.

Sloppy Joes ●

Here's a meal that is great for lunch and dinner. It hits home for the whole family on a cold winter night or after a weekend hockey game. Serve it with freshly cut veggies and hummus for dipping. Choose a whole-wheat pita half to serve it with and top it off with a sprinkling of chopped lettuce and tomato.

> 1 pound extra-lean ground beef
> 1 onion, chopped
> 4 cloves garlic, minced
> 1 green bell pepper, stemmed, seeded, and chopped
> ½ jalapeño pepper, stemmed, seeded, and minced
> 1 can (19 ounces) kidney beans, drained and rinsed
> 1 can (28 ounces) diced tomatoes
> ¼ cup old-fashioned rolled oats
> 1 tablespoon chili powder
> 2 teaspoons Worcestershire sauce
> 4 whole-wheat pita halves
> 2 cups chopped romaine or iceberg lettuce
> 2 tomatoes, chopped

1. Cook the beef in a large, deep nonstick skillet or Dutch o medium-high heat until browned, about 8 minutes. Add the onion, garlic, bell pepper, and jalapeño pepper and cook for 5 minutes. Add the beans, tomatoes, oats, chili powder, and Worcestershire sauce and bring to a boil. Reduce the heat and simmer, stirring occasionally, until thickened, about 25 minutes.

2. Scoop the sloppy joe mixture into pita halves and top with lettuce and tomato.

(continued)

Poultry Option:
You can use ground turkey or chicken instead of beef.

Vegetarian Option:
You can use ground meat substitute instead of the beef.

Chili Option:
This can be eaten like a chili. Simply reduce the cooking time to about 15 minutes for a chili consistency.

Classic Meat Lasagna ●

8 servings

Cheese is a favorite part of lasagna that adds a creamy, gooey layer. You can get that gooey rich flavor with a béchamel sauce, instead of ricotta cheese. By adding more veggies to the meat mixture we bulk it up with flavor and fiber.

1 pound extra-lean ground beef or veal
1 onion, finely chopped
4 cloves garlic, minced
8 ounces mushrooms, sliced
2 zucchini, trimmed and chopped
1 red bell pepper, stemmed, seeded, and chopped
1 green bell pepper, stemmed, seeded,
    and chopped
1 tablespoon dried oregano
½ teaspoon red pepper flakes
½ cup beef broth (low-fat, low-sodium)
2 cans (28 ounces each) tomato puree
Salt

¼ *teaspoon black pepper*
12 *whole-wheat lasagna noodles*

Béchamel Sauce
¼ *cup canola oil*
½ *cup whole-wheat flour*
4 *cups warm skim milk*
2 *tablespoons grated Parmesan cheese*
¼ *teaspoon salt*
¼ *teaspoon black pepper*
Pinch of nutmeg

1. Cook the ground beef, onion, and garlic in a large, shallow Dutch oven or deep nonstick skillet over medium heat until browned, about 8 minutes. Add the mushrooms, zucchini, bell peppers, oregano, and red pepper flakes and cook, stirring occasionally, until the onion has softened, about 10 minutes. Add the broth and bring to a boil. Cook until all the liquid has evaporated, then add the tomato puree, ¼ teaspoon of salt, and black pepper and bring to a boil again. Reduce the heat and simmer until thickened, about 30 minutes.

2. Bring a large pot of salted water to a boil.

3. *Make the Béchamel Sauce:* Heat the oil in a saucepan over medium-high heat. Add the flour and cook, stirring, for 1 minute. Slowly pour in the milk and whisk to combine. Cook, whisking gently, until the mixture is thick enough to coat the back of a spoon, about 5 minutes. Add the cheese, salt, pepper, and nutmeg. Remove from the heat.

4. Meanwhile, cook the lasagna noodles in the boiling water until al dente, about 10 minutes. Drain, and rinse under cold water. Lay the noodles flat on damp tea towels and set aside.

(continued)

5. Preheat the oven to 350°F.

6. Ladle 1½ cups of the meat sauce into the bottom of a 9 × 13-inch glass baking dish. Lay 3 noodles side by side on top of the sauce. Spread with another 1 cup of the meat sauce, then ¼ of the béchamel sauce. Repeat the layers (noodles, meat sauce, béchamel sauce) ending with béchamel sauce. Cover the dish with aluminum foil and place it on a baking sheet to catch any drips. Bake for 45 minutes, then uncover and bake for 15 minutes, or until bubbly and a knife inserted in the center is hot to the touch. Cool 10 minutes before serving.

Storage:
You can assemble the lasagna and refrigerate it for up to 1 day before baking. You can also freeze the baked lasagna whole or in portions and reheat it in the oven or microwave.

Veal Parmesan ●

4 servings

Traditionally, this classic Italian dish is made with breaded, fried veal. I've lightened it up by omitting the bread crumbs and grilling the veal instead. Tuscan White Bean Soup (page 121) makes a perfect starter with this dish.

> *2 tablespoons grated Parmesan cheese*
> *1½ teaspoons Italian herb seasoning*
> *½ teaspoon salt*
> *½ teaspoon black pepper*

1 pound veal, cut into 4 slices and pounded thin,
*   or leg cutlets*
1 cup low-fat tomato sauce, heated
¼ cup shredded part-skim mozzarella cheese
2 tablespoons chopped fresh flat-leaf parsley or basil

1. Preheat an outdoor grill or a grill pan.

2. Combine the Parmesan cheese, Italian herb seasoning, salt, and pepper in a small bowl. Sprinkle the mixture on both sides of the veal scallopini.

3. Place the veal on the greased grill over high heat. Close the lid and grill, turning once, for about 5 minutes, or until no longer pink inside. Place the grilled veal in a shallow dish, pour the sauce over the top, and sprinkle with the mozzarella and parsley.

Skillet Option:
If a grill is unavailable, you can cook the cutlets in a nonstick skillet with 2 teaspoons of extra-virgin olive oil.

Vegetarian Option:
You can use 1 eggplant, cut into ½-inch-thick slices, instead of the veal. Brush the slices with 1 tablespoon extra-virgin olive oil, then sprinkle with the seasoning mixture. Grill over medium-high heat for 20 minutes, or until tender, turning once, and serve with the sauce as above.

Hearty Veal Stew ●

6 servings

This is one of my favorite recipes to make on the weekend. Long cooking makes the veal melt in your mouth. You can also try beef or pork with this recipe.

> *1½ pounds lean boneless veal shoulder*
> *2 tablespoons whole-wheat flour*
> *2 teaspoons Italian herb seasoning*
> *½ teaspoon salt*
> *½ teaspoon black pepper*
> *2 tablespoons canola oil*
> *2 onions, sliced*
> *4 cloves garlic, minced*
> *1 stalk celery, chopped*
> *1 carrot, chopped*
> *3 cups beef broth (low-fat, low-sodium)*
> *¼ cup tomato paste*
> *1 tablespoon Worcestershire sauce*
> *1 can (15 ounces) cannellini beans, drained and rinsed*
> *1 cup snow peas, halved*

1. Trim the veal of any visible fat and cut it into 1-inch cubes. Set aside.

2. Combine the flour, Italian herb seasoning, salt, and pepper in a shallow dish or pie plate. Toss the veal with the flour mixture to coat.

3. Heat the oil in a large, shallow pot over medium-high heat. Add the veal in batches and cook, turning the pieces to brown all sides, then remove to a plate. Reduce the heat to medium and add the onions, garlic, celery, carrot, and any remaining flour mixture. Cook until the onions start to turn golden, about 5 minutes. Add the broth, tomato paste, and Worcestershire sauce. Bring to a boil and return the veal to the pot.

4. Reduce the heat to low, cover, and simmer for 1 hour, or until the veal is tender. Uncover, and add the beans and snow peas. Cook for another 15 minutes, or until the snow peas are tender-crisp.

Veal with Fennel and Mushrooms ●

4 servings

Veal is a lean and tender cut and is wonderful paired with the aromatic flavor of fennel. Fennel, also called anise, can be found in the produce section of your grocery store and has a mild licorice flavor.

1 pound veal, cut into 4 slices
¾ teaspoon salt
½ teaspoon black pepper
1 tablespoon extra-virgin olive oil
1 pound mushrooms, sliced
½ fennel bulb, trimmed and thinly sliced
2 tablespoons chopped fresh sage or 2 teaspoons dried
½ cup dry white or Marsala wine
¼ cup chopped fresh flat-leaf parsley

(continued)

1. Using a meat pounder, pound the slices of veal to ⅛-inch thickness. Sprinkle with ½ teaspoon of the salt and the pepper.

2. Heat half of the oil in a large nonstick skillet over medium-high heat. Add the veal in batches and cook, for 2 minutes per side, or until browned. Remove to a plate and keep warm.

3. Return the skillet to the heat and add the remaining oil. Add the mushrooms, fennel, sage, and remaining salt and cook for 15 minutes, or until all the liquid has evaporated and the mushrooms are beginning to brown. Add the wine and boil for 3 minutes. Pour the sauce over the veal and sprinkle with parsley before serving.

Veal Piccata Option:
Instead of using wine, you can substitute ¼ cup lemon juice and ½ teaspoon of grated lemon zest and boil for 1 minute. Add 1 tablespoon of chopped capers.

Chunky Lamb and Bean Stew

4 servings

The beans in this dish provide a creamy sauce for the lamb. This classic combination could become one of your family's new favorites.

> *1½ pounds lean boneless lamb*
> *1 tablespoon canola oil*
> *2 onions, chopped*
> *2 cloves garlic, minced*
> *1 tablespoon chopped fresh thyme leaves or*
>   *1 teaspoon dried*

2 teaspoons chopped fresh rosemary or
  ½ teaspoon dried
½ teaspoon red pepper flakes
½ teaspoon salt
½ teaspoon black pepper
3 cups beef broth (low-fat, low-sodium)
1 bay leaf
1 can (19 ounces) cannellini beans, drained and rinsed
1 tomato, chopped
¼ cup chopped fresh flat-leaf parsley

1. Cut the lamb into ½-inch cubes. Heat the oil in a large, shallow saucepan over medium-high heat. Add the lamb in batches and cook, stirring, until browned on all sides. Remove to a plate.

2. Reduce the heat to medium and add the onions, garlic, thyme, rosemary, red pepper flakes, salt, and pepper. Cook until the onions have softened, about 5 minutes. Add the broth, bay leaf, and browned lamb to the onion mixture and bring to a boil. Cover, reduce the heat to low, and simmer for 1 hour.

3. Meanwhile, put the beans in a large, shallow bowl and with a potato masher, coarsely mash them. Add the beans, tomato, and parsley to the lamb, cover, and continue cooking for about 30 minutes, or until the lamb is very tender and the sauce is thickened. Remove the bay leaf.

Pork Tenderloin with Grainy Mustard and Chive Crust ●

3 servings

Pork is a very lean meat and is delicious when paired with mustard. Try different kinds such as Dijon or herb-flavored mustard for variety. Serve this with carrots, broccoli, and couscous for a quick but elegant dinner.

> *1 pork tenderloin (12 ounces)*
> *¼ cup grainy mustard*
> *1 clove garlic, minced*
> *2 tablespoons chopped fresh chives or scallions*
> *1 teaspoon canola oil*

1. Preheat the oven to 425°F.

2. Using a sharp knife, trim any excess fat and silverskin from the tenderloin.

3. Combine the mustard, garlic, chives, and oil in a small bowl. Spread this mixture evenly over the pork tenderloin. Place the tenderloin on a small baking sheet lined with parchment paper or aluminum foil. Roast for about 18 minutes, or until just a hint of pink remains inside.

4. Place the tenderloin under the broiler for 1 minute to brown, turn, and repeat with the other side. Let stand for 5 minutes before thinly slicing.

Pork Tenderloin with Apple Compote ●

3 servings

S erve this comforting dish with Brussels sprouts, sliced carrots, and some boiled new potatoes tossed in lemon juice and parsley.

1 tablespoon Dijon mustard
½ teaspoon dried sage leaves
¼ teaspoon dried thyme leaves
Pinch of salt
Pinch of black pepper
1 pork tenderloin (12-ounces), trimmed of fat
1 tablespoon canola oil

Apple Compote
1 teaspoon canola oil
2 small apples, cored and diced
1 onion, finely chopped
¼ teaspoon dried thyme leaves
Pinch of salt
Pinch of black pepper
¼ cup currants
2 tablespoons apple juice

1. Preheat the oven to 400°F.

2. In a small bowl, stir together the mustard, sage, thyme, salt, and pepper. Rub the mixture all over the tenderloin.

3. Heat the oil in an ovenproof nonstick skillet over medium-high heat. Brown the tenderloin on one side, then turn it over and place

(continued)

the skillet in the oven for about 20 minutes, or until the pork has only a hint of pink inside. Let stand for 5 minutes before slicing.

4. *Meanwhile, make the Apple Compote:* In another nonstick skillet, heat the oil over medium-high heat. Add the apples, onion, thyme, salt, and pepper and cook for 5 minutes, or until the apples are light golden. Add the currants and apple juice and cook for 1 minute more, just until the apples are tender-crisp. Slice the tenderloin and serve with the compote.

Pork Amandine

2 servings

This meal can be ready faster than it takes to set the table! Serve with a big helping of steamed green beans or asparagus.

> *4 boneless pork loin chops (4 ounces each), trimmed*
> *of fat and pounded to ⅛-inch thickness*
> *1 clove garlic, minced*
> *¼ teaspoon dried thyme leaves*
> *Pinch of salt*
> *Pinch of black pepper*
> *1 teaspoon canola oil*
> *¼ cup dry white wine*
> *¼ cup chicken broth (low-fat, low-sodium)*
> *½ teaspoon cornstarch dissolved in 2 teaspoons water*
> *2 tablespoons toasted sliced almonds (see Note)*
> *1 tablespoon chopped fresh flat-leaf parsley*

1. Sprinkle both sides of each pork chop with the garlic, thyme, salt, and pepper. Heat the oil in a large nonstick skillet over medium-high heat. Cook the chops, turning once, until browned, about 5 minutes. Remove to a plate.

2. Return the skillet to medium-high heat and add the wine and broth. Bring to a boil and cook for 1 minute. Add the cornstarch mixture and cook, stirring, for 30 seconds. Return the pork chops to the pan, turning to coat. Sprinkle with almonds and parsley before serving.

Chicken Stock Option:
If you don't want to use wine in this recipe, simply use the same amount of chicken broth. Stir in 1 teaspoon lemon juice to add some tang to the sauce.

Note:
To toast raw almonds, heat a dry skillet over medium heat. Add the almonds and, shaking the pan frequently, toast until they are just starting to turn golden, about 5 minutes.

Pesto Pork Chops

4 servings

This is a quick and easy dinner to put on the table during a busy work week.

> 4 boneless pork loin chops, trimmed of fat
> ¼ cup pesto
> ¼ teaspoon salt
> ¼ teaspoon black pepper
> 1 teaspoon canola oil
> 1 onion, sliced
> 1 red bell pepper, stemmed, seeded, and thinly sliced
> ½ teaspoon dried oregano
> ⅓ cup chicken broth (low-fat, low-sodium)

1. In a nonstick skillet, over medium-high heat, cook the pork chops, turning once, until brown on both sides. Remove to a plate. Spread the pesto over the chops and sprinkle with half each of the salt and black pepper. Set aside.

2. In the same skillet, add the oil, onion, bell pepper, oregano, and remaining salt and black pepper. Cook, stirring, over medium-high heat until the onion turns golden, about 4 minutes. Add the broth and pork chops, pesto side up. Cover, and continue cooking until the pork chops have just a hint of pink inside, about 5 minutes.

Green-Light Chicken Option:
You can use 4 boneless, skinless chicken breasts or 8 boneless, skinless chicken thighs instead of the pork chops.

Pesto Option:
Look for sun-dried tomato pesto in your grocery store and use it in this recipe for a new taste.

Apple Pork Chops

4 servings

For this dish, choose a cooking apple such as Crispin, Golden Delicious, or Northern Spy. The lovely sauce goes very well with basmati rice.

> *4 boneless pork loin chops, trimmed of fat*
> *½ teaspoon salt*
> *Pinch of black pepper*
> *1 teaspoon canola oil*
> *2 apples, cored and sliced*
> *1 large onion, sliced*
> *1 cup water*
> *2 tablespoons raisins*
> *1 bay leaf*
> *1½ teaspoons blackstrap molasses*
> *1½ teaspoons cider vinegar*
> *¼ teaspoon dried thyme leaves*
> *2 teaspoons cornstarch*

1. Sprinkle the porkchops on both sides with half each of the salt and the pepper.

2. In a large nonstick skillet over medium-high heat, heat the oil. Add the chops and cook, turning once, until brown on both sides. Top the chops with the apples and onion. Pour in all but 2 tablespoons of the water. Add the raisins, bay leaf, molasses, vinegar, thyme, and remaining salt and pepper and bring to a boil. Cover, reduce the heat, and simmer for about 45 minutes, or until the pork is tender.

3. In a small bowl, whisk together the cornstarch and reserved water. Add to the skillet and cook, stirring, until the sauce is slightly thickened, about 1 minute. Remove the bay leaf.

Apricot–Sage Stuffed Pork Chops

4 servings

These pork chops are wonderful entertaining fare. Serve with green beans and carrots tossed with a touch of extra-virgin olive oil and garlic.

> *3 teaspoons canola oil*
> *1 small onion, minced*
> *2 cloves garlic, minced*
> *2 tablespoons chopped fresh sage leaves or*
> *   2 teaspoons dried*
> *½ red bell pepper, stemmed, seeded, and diced*
> *1 cup fresh whole-wheat bread crumbs*
> *¼ cup diced dried apricots*
> *¼ cup chopped fresh flat-leaf parsley*
> *⅓ cup liquid egg*
> *Salt and black pepper*
> *4 thick, boneless pork loin chops,*
> *   trimmed of fat*

1. *Make the stuffing:* Heat 1 teaspoon of the oil in a nonstick skillet over medium heat. Add the onion, garlic, sage, and bell pepper and cook until the onion has softened, about 6 minutes. Stir in the bread crumbs, apricots, and parsley and remove from the heat. Stir in the liquid egg, ¼ teaspoon salt, and ¼ teaspoon black pepper until well combined. Set aside.

2. In each pork chop cut a pocket almost all the way through, leaving one long side attached, and open the chop up like a book. Spoon one fourth of the stuffing on one side of each chop and fold the other side of the meat over the stuffing. Sprinkle with a pinch of salt and pepper.

3. Preheat the oven to 425°F.

4. In a nonstick skillet over medium-high heat, heat the remaining 2 teaspoons of oil. Brown the pork chops on both sides. Place the chops on a baking sheet lined with parchment paper or aluminum foil and roast for about 20 minutes, or until just a hint of pink remains in the center of the pork.

Green-Light Chicken Option:
You can use 4 boneless, skinless chicken breasts instead of the pork chops.

Artichoke and Pork Stew

6 servings

Canned artichokes need a good rinse before use to remove the brine flavor. Serve this stew over rice alongside mesclun greens tossed with balsamic vinegar and pepper.

> *1½ pounds boneless pork loin chops, trimmed of fat*
> *2 tablespoons whole-wheat flour*
> *1 teaspoon ground cumin*
> *¼ teaspoon ground turmeric*
> *¼ teaspoon ground coriander*
> *¼ teaspoon salt*
> *Pinch of ground cinnamon*
> *Pinch of ground cloves*
> *1 tablespoon canola oil, plus more if needed*
> *1 cup chicken broth (low-fat, low-sodium) or water*
> *2 onions, chopped*
> *2 cloves garlic, minced*
> *1 carrot, chopped*
> *1 green bell pepper, stemmed, seeded, and chopped*
> *1 can (28 ounces) diced tomatoes*
> *2 jars (6.5 ounces each) artichoke hearts, drained,*
> *   rinsed, and quartered*
> *1 cup frozen peas*

1. Cut the pork chops into ½-inch-thick strips and set aside. Combine the flour, cumin, turmeric, coriander, salt, cinnamon, and cloves in a shallow dish or pie plate. Toss the pork strips with the flour mixture to coat.

2. Heat the oil in a large shallow pot over medium-high heat. Working in batches, add the pork and cook until browned, adding more oil if necessary. Remove the cooked pork to a plate. Add the broth to the pot and scrape up the brown bits, stirring constantly. Add the onions, garlic, carrot, and bell pepper and cook for 5 minutes. Add the tomatoes and bring to a boil. Return the meat and its juices to the pan, reduce the heat, cover, and simmer for about 1 hour, or until the pork is tender.

3. Add the artichokes and peas and cook, uncovered, for 15 minutes, or until slightly thickened.

SNACKS

Dried Chickpeas ●

3 cups

This is an addictive snack with all the crunch and saltiness of chips and pretzels but without the fat!

> *2 cans (15 ounces each) chickpeas, drained and rinsed*
> *2 tablespoons extra-virgin olive oil or canola oil*
> *½ teaspoon salt (see Hint)*
> *Pinch of cayenne pepper*

1. Preheat the oven to 400°F.

2. Toss the chickpeas in a large bowl with the oil, salt, and cayenne. Spread onto a large baking sheet in a single layer.

3. Bake, shaking the pan a couple of times during cooking, for about 45 minutes, or until golden. Let cool completely.

Helpful Hint:
You can add more salt or other spices if you would like to change the flavor of the chickpeas.

Sage and Tomato
White Bean Dip ●

1 1/2 cups

I like to serve this at parties with vegetables and whole-wheat pita crisps. It's also great smeared over a turkey sandwich.

2 tablespoons chopped sun-dried tomatoes
1/4 cup boiling water
1 can (15 ounces) cannellini beans, drained and rinsed
2 tablespoons extra-virgin olive oil
1/2 teaspoon salt
Pinch of black pepper
1 tablespoon chopped fresh sage leaves or
   1/2 teaspoon dried
1 small clove garlic, minced

1. Place the sun-dried tomatoes in the boiling water and let them stand for 10 minutes. Drain, and reserve the water.

2. In a food processor, puree the beans, sun-dried tomatoes, oil, salt, pepper, and 2 tablespoons of the reserved water until smooth. Pulse in the sage and garlic.

Storage:
Keep in an airtight container, refrigerated, for up to 2 weeks.

Roasted Red Pepper Hummus ●

1 1/2 cups

S erve this as a dip with raw veggies or as a spread for sandwiches or hamburgers. You could also enjoy it on its own in half a whole-wheat pita with tomatoes and cucumber slices.

> *1 can (15 ounces) chickpeas, drained and rinsed*
> *1/2 cup chopped roasted red peppers*
> *1/4 cup tahini (see Hint)*
> *1/2 teaspoon ground cumin*
> *1/2 teaspoon salt*
> *2 tablespoons extra-virgin olive oil*
> *2 tablespoons water*
> *1 tablespoon fresh lemon juice*
> *1 small clove garlic, minced*

In a food processor, pulse together the chickpeas, peppers, tahini, cumin, and salt. With the food processor running, add the oil and water and blend until very smooth. Pulse in the lemon juice and garlic.

Storage:
Keep in an airtight container, refrigerated, for up to 2 weeks.

Sun-Dried Tomato Option:
Omit the roasted red peppers. Replace with 1/4 cup of chopped sun-dried tomatoes that have been rehydrated in hot water and drained.

Roasted Vegetable Option:
Omit the roasted red peppers. Replace with 1/2 cup of other chopped roasted vegetables.

Helpful Hint:
Tahini is a sesame-seed paste that you can find in most grocery stores. You can also find it in health and bulk food stores. It adds a great nutty flavor to the hummus.

Over-the-Top Bran Muffins
with Pears ●

12 muffins

These muffins are big and full of fiber. They are over-the-top because they rise above the top of the pan, so be sure to grease the top of your muffin pan too! The addition of chopped fresh pear keeps the muffins moist. These muffins are great alongside a cup of decaf or a glass of milk in the morning and perfect, too, for an afternoon pick-me-up at the office.

1 cup All-Bran or 100% Bran cereal
1 cup wheat bran
1½ cups plain low-fat yogurt
2 cups whole-wheat flour
½ cup brown sugar substitute
1 tablespoon baking powder
2 teaspoons baking soda
¼ teaspoon salt
½ cup skim milk
¼ cup canola oil
1 egg
2 teaspoons vanilla extract
2 pears, cored and diced

1. Combine the cereal and wheat bran in a bowl. Stir in the yogurt and let stand for 10 minutes.

2. In a separate bowl, combine the flour, brown sugar substitute, baking powder, baking soda, and salt.

(continued)

3. Add the milk, oil, egg, and vanilla to the bran mixture and stir to combine. Pour over the flour mixture and stir until just combined. Stir in the pears.

4. Preheat the oven to 375°F.

5. Divide the batter among 12 greased or paper-lined muffin cups. Bake until the tops are golden and firm to the touch, about 25 minutes. Let cool on a rack for 5 minutes. Remove the muffins from the pan and let cool completely.

Storage:
Keep covered at room temperature for about 2 days, or frozen for up to 1 month. To freeze, wrap each muffin individually, then place them in a resealable plastic bag or airtight container.

Dried Fruit Option:
Use 1 cup dried cranberries, raisins, diced apricots, or dried blueberries instead of the pear.

Blueberry Option:
Use 2 cups fresh blueberries instead of the pear.

Whole-Wheat Scones ●

8 scones

I love these scones with a hot cup of tea in the afternoon. The sweet fruit version makes a wonderful breakfast treat when topped with a little low-sugar fruit spread.

> *1 ½ cups whole-wheat flour*
> *½ cup oat bran*
> *3 scallions, chopped*
> *3 tablespoons flax or sunflower seeds*
> *2 teaspoons baking powder*
> *2 teaspoons sugar substitute*
> *½ teaspoon salt*
> *¼ teaspoon ground nutmeg*
> *¼ cup nonhydrogenated soft margarine*
> *⅔ cup skim milk*
> *2 tablespoons liquid egg*

1. In a large bowl, combine the flour, oat bran, scallions, flax seeds, baking powder, sugar substitute, salt, and nutmeg. Use your fingers to rub the margarine into the flour mixture to combine. Add the milk and stir with a fork to make a soft dough.

2. Preheat the oven to 425°F.

3. Place the dough on a floured surface and knead gently about 5 times. Pat the dough out to a ½-inch thickness and cut it into 8 squares. (Alternatively, you can use a cookie or biscuit cutter to cut round scones.) Place the scones on an ungreased baking sheet and brush the tops with liquid egg. Bake until golden on the bottom, about 12 minutes.

(continued)

Sweet Fruit Option:
Omit the scallions and flax seeds. Increase the sugar substitute to
2 tablespoons and add ½ cup chopped dried apricots, raisins, or
dried cranberries.

Orange Bran Muffins

12 muffins

My wife makes this recipe to raves from our friends. Though it
calls for a whole orange, the sugar substitute removes the
bitterness of the rind. Use a navel orange, which has no seeds and
is very juicy.

> *1 whole navel orange*
> *¾ cup skim milk*
> *½ cup fresh orange juice*
> *¼ cup nonhydrogenated soft margarine*
> *1 egg*
> *1 teaspoon vanilla extract*
> *2 cups whole-wheat flour*
> *½ cup wheat bran*
> *¼ cup sugar substitute*
> *1 teaspoon baking powder*
> *1 teaspoon baking soda*
> *1 teaspoon ground cinnamon*
> *Pinch of salt*

1. Cut the orange into 8 wedges. Place in a food processor and
pulse until finely chopped or almost pureed. Add the milk, orange
juice, margarine, egg, and vanilla and pulse until combined.

2. Preheat the oven to 400°F.

3. In a large bowl, combine the flour, bran, sugar substitute, baking powder, baking soda, cinnamon, and salt. Pour the orange mixture over the flour mixture and stir until just combined. Divide the batter among 12 greased or paper-lined muffin cups. Bake until golden and firm to the touch, about 20 minutes.

Storage:
Keep covered at room temperature for about 2 days, or frozen for up to 1 month. To freeze, wrap each muffin individually, then place them in a resealable plastic bag or airtight container.

Cranberry Cinnamon Bran Muffins ●

12 muffins

These muffins are very nutritious—they have a high fiber content—and are redolent of cinnamon.

> *1 cup wheat bran*
> *½ cup All-Bran or 100% Bran cereal*
> *¼ teaspoon salt*
> *½ cup boiling water*
> *1 cup skim milk*
> *1 cup dried cranberries*
> *⅓ cup sugar substitute*
> *1 egg*
> *¼ cup canola oil*
> *1¼ cups whole-wheat flour*
> *1¼ teaspoons baking soda*
> *1 teaspoon ground cinnamon*

1. Combine the wheat bran, cereal, and salt in a bowl. Add the boiling water and stir to combine. Stir in the milk and cranberries and set aside.

2. In another bowl, whisk together the sugar substitute, egg, and oil. Stir into the bran mixture.

3. Preheat the oven to 375°F.

4. In a third, large bowl, stir together the flour, baking soda, and cinnamon. Pour the bran mixture over the flour mixture and stir until just combined. Divide the batter among 12 lined or greased muffin cups. Bake for about 20 minutes, or until a cake tester inserted in the center comes out clean.

Storage:
Store, covered, at room temperature for about 2 days or frozen for up to 1 month. To freeze, wrap each muffin individually, then place them in a resealable plastic bag or airtight container.

Lemon Blueberry Muffins

9 muffins

L emon and blueberries have a natural affinity for each other, as these delicious muffins prove.

> 1 ½ cups whole-wheat flour
> ½ cup wheat bran
> ½ cup sugar substitute
> 1 tablespoon baking powder
> ½ teaspoon salt
> 1 cup skim milk
> 1 egg
> ¼ cup nonhydrogenated soft margarine, melted,
>   or canola oil
> 1 tablespoon grated lemon zest
> 1 cup fresh or frozen blueberries

1. Combine the flour, wheat bran, sugar substitute, baking powder, and salt in a large bowl. In another, smaller bowl, whisk together the milk, egg, margarine, and lemon zest. Pour the milk mixture over the flour mixture and stir until just combined. Stir in the blueberries.

2. Preheat the oven to 375°F.

(continued)

3. Divide the batter among 9 lined or greased muffin cups. Fill the empty muffin cups about ⅔ full of water to prevent the pan from burning. Bake for about 20 minutes, or until golden and firm to the touch.

Storage:
These muffins can be kept at room temperature for about 2 days or frozen for up to 3 weeks. To freeze, wrap each muffin individually, then place them in a resealable plastic bag or airtight container.

Helpful Hint:
If using frozen blueberries, do not thaw. Add them directly to the batter.

Apple Raisin Bread

1 loaf

A slice of this bread makes a delicious afternoon snack. You can also toast it and top it with a little margarine.

> 1 ¼ cups whole-wheat flour
> ½ cup wheat bran
> ½ cup sugar substitute
> 2 teaspoons ground cinnamon
> 1 teaspoon baking powder
> ½ teaspoon baking soda
> ¼ teaspoon ground nutmeg
> ¼ teaspoon salt
> 2 apples, cored and diced
> ⅓ cup raisins

⅓ *cup chopped pecans or almonds (optional)*
1 *cup buttermilk (see Hint)*
⅓ *cup liquid egg*
¼ *cup canola oil*
2 *tablespoons brown sugar substitute (optional)*

1. Combine the flour, wheat bran, sugar substitute, cinnamon, baking powder, baking soda, nutmeg, and salt in a large bowl. Toss in the apples, raisins, and pecans (if using) to coat them with flour.

2. Preheat the oven to 350°F.

3. In a smaller bowl, whisk together the buttermilk, liquid egg, and oil. Pour over the flour mixture and stir until just combined. Pour the batter into a 5 × 9-inch greased loaf pan. Sprinkle the top with brown sugar substitute if you like. Bake for about 45 minutes, or until golden and a cake tester inserted in the center comes out clean. Let cool on a rack.

Storage:
Keep wrapped in plastic wrap and aluminum foil for 3 days. The bread also freezes well for up to 1 month.

Helpful Hint:
You don't have buttermilk in your refrigerator? No problem. Substitute 1 tablespoon of lemon juice or white vinegar mixed with 1 cup of skim milk. Let stand a couple of minutes.

Blueberry Bars ●

24 bars

This is a spin off of a breakfast bar but it contains much more fiber and many fewer calories. You can make these bars on the weekend and eat them through the week at snack time.

> *2 ½ cups frozen blueberries*
> *¼ cup water*
> *2 tablespoons sugar substitute*
> *½ teaspoon grated lemon zest*
> *2 teaspoons fresh lemon juice*
> *1 tablespoon cornstarch*
> *1 cup old-fashioned rolled oats*
> *¾ cup whole-wheat flour*
> *¾ cup wheat bran*
> *½ cup brown sugar substitute*
> *¼ teaspoon baking soda*
> *½ cup soft nonhydrogenated margarine*
> *3 tablespoons liquid egg*

1. Bring the blueberries, water, sugar substitute, lemon zest and juice, and cornstarch to a boil in a saucepan over medium heat. Cook, stirring, until thickened and bubbly, about 2 minutes. Let cool.

2. Preheat the oven to 350°F.

3. Combine the oats, flour, wheat bran, brown sugar substitute, and baking soda in a bowl. Use a wooden spoon to work in the margarine until the mixture resembles coarse crumbs. Add the liquid egg and stir until moistened. Reserve ¾ cup of the mixture for the top. Press the remaining mixture into the bottom of an 8-inch square baking pan lined with parchment paper. Spread with blueberry filling. Sprinkle with the reserved oat mixture.

4. Bake until the crust is golden and the blueberry filling is bubbly at the edges, about 30 minutes. Let cool completely before cutting into bars.

Storage:
Place the bars in an airtight container and keep refrigerated for up to 5 days or freeze for up to 2 weeks.

Almond Bran Haystacks ●

18 cookies

These cookies are best the day they are baked. After that they tend to lose their crispness, though they still taste yummy. Enjoy them with a cup of decaf coffee or skim milk.

2 egg whites
¼ teaspoon cream of tartar
⅓ cup sugar substitute
1 ¼ cups All-Bran or 100% Bran cereal
½ cup chopped toasted almonds
1 tablespoon vanilla extract
¼ teaspoon almond extract

1. Beat the egg whites and cream of tartar in a large bowl until soft peaks form. Gradually add the sugar substitute and beat until stiff peaks form. Fold in the cereal, almonds, vanilla, and almond extract until combined.

2. Preheat the oven to 325°F.

3. Drop the batter by tablespoonfuls onto a baking sheet lined with parchment paper. Bake until lightly browned and firm to the touch, about 15 minutes. Let cool completely.

Storage:
Keep in an airtight container for up to 5 days. These do not freeze well.

Oatcakes ●

16 oatcakes

Scottish oatcakes have been around for a long time. These taste delicious on their own or alongside a cup of tea. Traditionally they were made without sweetening, but over time the sweetened version appeared and people got hooked. You can try them without the sugar substitute and see which you prefer.

> 2 cups old-fashioned rolled oats
> 1 cup whole-wheat flour
> ½ cup wheat bran
> 1 tablespoon wheat germ
> ⅓ cup sugar substitute
> ½ teaspoon salt
> ½ cup nonhydrogenated soft margarine
> 1 egg, lightly beaten
> 3 tablespoons water

1. Combine the oats, flour, wheat bran and germ, sugar substitute, and salt in a large bowl. Use a wooden spoon to stir in the margarine until a crumbly mixture forms. Add the egg and water and stir until the dough sticks together.

2. Preheat the oven to 350°F.

3. Divide the dough into 16 pieces. Form each piece into a ¼-inch-thick round and place on a baking sheet lined with parchment paper. Bake for 15 minutes. Turn the oatcakes over and bake on the other side until firm and golden, about 10 minutes.

Storage:
Keep in a plastic resealable bag or airtight container for 5 days or in the freezer for up to 3 weeks.

Fresh Fruit Bowl ●

4 cups; 4 servings

K eep this in the fridge and have a bowl for an afternoon snack or
after-dinner pick-me-up.

> *2 oranges*
> *2 kiwis, peeled and sliced*
> *2 nectarines, pitted and sliced*
> *1 star fruit, sliced (optional)*
> *1 cup trimmed, halved strawberries*
> *1 cup red or green seedless grapes*
> *1 cup blueberries or raspberries*
> *1 tablespoon sugar substitute*
> *1 teaspoon fresh lemon juice*
> *Pinch of ground ginger*

1. Using a serrated knife, cut both ends off the oranges. Using a
sawing motion, cut off the peel and pith. Over a large bowl, cut the
oranges into sections, discarding the membranes but reserving as
much juice as possible. Set aside.

2. Add the kiwis, nectarines, star fruit (if desired), strawberries,
grapes, and blueberries to the oranges. Toss to combine.

3. Sprinkle the sugar substitute, lemon juice, and ginger over the
fruit and toss to combine.

Storage:
Cover and refrigerate for up to 2 days.

Serving Option:
You can sprinkle the fruit with sliced almonds and serve with a
dollop of yogurt, if desired.

SIDE DISHES AND BASICS

Classic Cooked Vegetables ●

Vegetables are delicious, inexpensive, and filled with vitamins and minerals, and almost all are green-light. Here is a list of my favorites with advice on how to prepare them for cooking, followed by instructions for three easy cooking methods. Once the vegetables are cooked, I dress them with a squeeze of lemon juice and a dash of salt and pepper or with my classic vinaigrette (page 133).

> *Asparagus: trim ends*
> *Broccoli: cut into florets*
> *Brussels sprouts: trim and halve*
> *Carrots: cut into ½-inch chunks*
> *Cauliflower: cut into florets*
> *Frozen green peas: do not thaw*
> *Frozen mixed vegetables: do not thaw*
> *Green beans: trim tips*
> *New potatoes: scrub and prick with fork*
> *Snow peas/sugar snap peas: trim tips*
> *Yellow beans: trim tips*
> *Zucchini: trim ends and cut into chunks*

1. *To boil:* Fill a saucepan with water and bring to a boil. Add the vegetable and cook until it is tender-crisp, about 2 to 10 minutes.

2. *To steam:* Fill a saucepan with water to a depth of 1 inch and bring to a boil. Place a steamer basket filled with the vegetable in the saucepan. Cover with the lid and steam until the vegetable is tender-crisp, 5 to 7 minutes.

3. *To microwave:* Place the vegetable in a large microwave-safe plate or bowl. Add ¼ cup of water. Cover with plastic wrap and microwave on High for about 5 minutes, or until the vegetable is tender-crisp.

White Bean Mash ●

4 servings

This creamy side dish is a higher-fiber option to mashed potatoes. The creaminess comes from the addition of chicken stock. Add watercress for a peppery bite or kale for a heartier winter version.

> *1 cup chicken broth (low-fat, low sodium)*
> *2 cans (19 ounces each) cannellini beans, drained*
>   *and rinsed*
> *¼ teaspoon dried thyme*
> *¼ teaspoon black pepper*
> *2 cups baby spinach leaves, shredded*
> *Pinch of salt*

1. Bring the broth to a boil in a saucepan. Add the beans, thyme, and pepper. Simmer for about 10 minutes.

2. Mash the bean mixture with a potato masher until fairly smooth. Stir in the spinach and salt until combined.

Baked Beans ●

8 servings

Normally, baked beans are packed with sugar and molasses, which adds lots of calories. Our version achieves the same comforting, filling, and fiber-packed effect without the sugar.

> 2 cups dry navy or small white beans
> 8 cups water
> 1 can (28 ounces) diced tomatoes
> 4 ounces lean Black Forest ham, chopped
> 1 large red onion, peeled and finely chopped
> 1 can (6 ounces) tomato paste
> ¼ cup brown sugar substitute
> 2 tablespoons Dijon mustard
> 1 tablespoon Worcestershire sauce
> 2 teaspoons Tabasco sauce
> ½ teaspoon salt
> ½ teaspoon black pepper

1. Rinse the beans and place them in a Dutch oven filled with water. Cover, and let soak overnight. The next day, drain and rinse the beans.

2. In the same pot, add the 8 cups of water and the beans and bring to a boil. Reduce the heat, cover, and simmer, stirring occasionally, for about 1½ hours, or until the beans are tender. Drain the beans, reserving the cooking liquid.

3. Preheat the oven to 300°F.

4. In a large bean pot or the same Dutch oven, combine 1 cup of the reserved cooking liquid, the beans, tomatoes, ham, onion, tomato paste, brown sugar substitute, mustard, Worcestershire sauce, Tabasco sauce, salt, and pepper. Cover, and bake, stirring occasionally, for 2½ hours. Uncover, and cook for 1 hour, or until thickened.

Quick-Soak Option:
Rinse the beans and place them in a Dutch oven filled with water. Bring to a boil and cook for 2 minutes. Cover, remove from the heat, and let sit for 1 hour. Then drain and continue with the recipe.

Slow-Cooker Option:
Place the cooked beans with the rest of the ingredients in a slow cooker and cook on Low for 8 to 10 hours or on High for 4 to 6 hours, or until tender.

Homemade Tomato Sauce ●

6 cups

My wife calls this tomato sauce the little black dress of the kitchen: It goes with everything. We use it in Easy-Bake Lasagna (page 180), Spaghetti and Meatballs (page 232), and Easy Meat Sauce (page 235). It takes just about an hour to make 6 cups so it has a very favorable effort–return ratio as well.

> 2 cans (26 ounces each) plum tomatoes
> 1 onion, chopped
> 2 cloves garlic, minced
> 1 zucchini, chopped
> 1 red bell pepper, stemmed, seeded, and chopped
> 2 teaspoons dried oregano
> ½ teaspoon salt
> ½ teaspoon black pepper

Place the tomatoes and their juices in a food processor and pulse until pureed. Transfer to a large saucepan and add the onion, garlic, zucchini, bell pepper, oregano, salt, and black pepper and bring to a boil. Turn the heat down to low and simmer, uncovered, until thickened slightly, about 40 minutes.

Storage:
Keep refrigerated for up to 1 week or freeze for up to 1 month.

Yogurt Cheese ●

1 ½ cups

This can be used as a tasty spread for whole-wheat toast, as a dip, or as a topping for a dessert (see Poached Pears, page 297). Yogurt cheese is also a great substitute for sour cream in most recipes.

24 ounces (3 cups) plain low-fat yogurt (see Note)

Line a sieve with cheesecloth and place it over a large bowl. Pour in the yogurt. Cover with plastic wrap, and refrigerate for at least 4 hours or overnight. Discard the liquid that has accumulated in the bowl. Remove the yogurt cheese from the sieve and use it right away or store it in an airtight container in the refrigerator.

Note:
Write down the "use-by" date on the container the yogurt came in, or keep the container. That's how long your yogurt cheese can be kept.

Sweet Yogurt Cheese:
Sweeten your yogurt cheese by adding sugar substitute to taste.

Lemony Yogurt Cheese:
Add 1 teaspoon of grated lemon zest and 2 teaspoons of fresh lemon juice along with sugar substitute to taste.

Quick Yogurt Cheese Dip:
Add 2 chopped scallions, 1 small minced garlic clove, 1 tablespoon of fresh lemon juice, and 1 tablespoon of chopped fresh oregano (or 1 teaspoon dried) to the yogurt cheese.

DESSERTS

Oatmeal Cookies ●

28 cookies

These soft, homey cookies are great as an after-lunch snack with a glass of milk. They are perfect for lunch bags, too. Kids and adults alike are always happy to get a cookie in their brown bags.

> *2 cups old-fashioned rolled oats*
> *¾ cup whole-wheat flour*
> *½ cup wheat bran*
> *½ teaspoon baking soda*
> *½ teaspoon ground cinnamon*
> *Pinch of salt*
> *1 cup brown sugar substitute*
> *½ cup nonhydrogenated soft margarine*
> *¼ cup liquid egg*
> *¼ cup water*
> *2 teaspoons vanilla extract*
> *½ cup dried currants (optional)*

1. In a large bowl, stir together the oats, flour, wheat bran, baking soda, cinnamon, and salt. Set aside.

2. In another large bowl, beat the brown sugar substitute, margarine, liquid egg, water, and vanilla until smooth. Stir the oat mixture into the margarine mixture until combined. Add the currants, if using, and stir to combine.

3. Preheat the oven to 375°F.

4. Drop the dough by heaping tablespoonfuls onto a baking sheet lined with parchment paper and flatten slightly. Bake until firm and golden on the bottom, about 8 minutes. Repeat with the remaining dough. Let cool on a rack.

Storage:
Keep in an airtight container for up to 3 days or freeze for up to 1 month.

Chewy Peanut Bars

12 bars

Here's a chewy granola treat that will be a favorite afternoon snack for the whole family.

> *1 ½ cups old-fashioned rolled oats*
> *¼ cup chopped unsalted peanuts (optional)*
> *½ cup wheat bran*
> *⅓ cup whole-wheat flour*
> *½ teaspoon baking soda*
> *½ teaspoon baking powder*
> *Pinch of salt*
> *Pinch of ground cinnamon*
> *⅔ cup liquid egg*
> *½ cup smooth peanut butter (natural, no sugar added)*
> *¼ cup brown sugar substitute*
> *2 teaspoons vanilla extract*

1. In a large bowl, combine the oats, peanuts (if using), wheat bran, flour, baking soda, baking powder, salt, and cinnamon.

(continued)

2. Preheat the oven to 350°F.

3. In another bowl, beat the liquid egg, peanut butter, brown sugar substitute, and vanilla until combined. Add the oat mixture and stir to combine. Scrape the dough into an 8-inch square baking pan lined with parchment paper. With damp hands, press down the mixture to flatten evenly.

4. Bake until firm to the touch, about 12 minutes. Let cool and cut into bars.

Storage:
Keep the bars wrapped individually with plastic wrap in an airtight container in the refrigerator for up to 4 days or freeze for up to 2 weeks.

Fruit Option:
Replace the peanuts with currants or dried cranberries.

Other Nut Butter Options:
If you don't feel like peanut butter, try replacing it with soy nut butter or almond or cashew butter, available in the organic section of the supermarket or health food store.

Chocolate Drop Cookies ●

24 cookies

These very moist cookies are great to eat warm and dunk into a glass of milk at snack time. You might be surprised to see beans in a dessert recipe, but trust us, they keep the batter tender and add fiber that kids don't even know they're getting. Sometimes it pays to be sneaky.

> ½ cup cooked cannellini beans
> 1 tablespoon wheat bran
> ¼ cup plus 2 tablespoons skim milk
> ⅓ cup nonhydrogenated soft margarine
> ¾ cup whole-wheat flour
> ½ cup sugar substitute
> ⅓ cup unsweetened cocoa powder
> 1 egg
> 2 teaspoons vanilla extract
> ½ teaspoon baking soda

1. Put the beans, wheat bran, and 2 tablespoons of the skim milk in a food processor and puree until well blended. Set aside.

2. Put the margarine, flour, sugar substitute, bean puree, cocoa powder, the remaining skim milk, the egg, vanilla, and baking soda in a bowl and beat until combined.

3. Preheat the oven to 375°F.

4. Drop the batter by tablespoonfuls onto a baking sheet lined with parchment paper. Bake until firm to the touch, about 10 minutes. Let cool on a rack.

Storage:
Keep in a resealable plastic bag or airtight container for about 3 days at room temperature or in the freezer for up to 3 weeks.

Chocolate Almond Slices ●

2 dozen cookies

These are similar to biscotti in that they are baked twice. Adults and kids love them and they are incredibly convenient—they keep well and are a perfect snack to take to the office or school. You could add ¼ cup of dried cranberries or raisins for some color and extra flavor if desired.

> *¼ cup nonhydrogenated soft margarine*
> *½ cup sugar substitute*
> *½ cup liquid egg*
> *4 teaspoons vanilla extract*
> *¼ teaspoon almond extract (optional)*
> *½ cup unsweetened cocoa powder*
> *½ cup wheat bran*
> *¼ cup wheat germ*
> *½ cup whole-wheat flour*
> *2 teaspoons baking powder*
> *Pinch of salt*
> *½ cup slivered almonds*

1. In a large bowl, cream together the margarine and sugar substitute. Beat in the liquid egg, vanilla, and almond extract, if using. Beat in the cocoa powder, wheat bran and germ, half of the flour, the baking powder, and salt. Stir in the remaining flour and knead in the almonds with your hands.

2. Preheat the oven to 350°F.

3. Shape the dough into 2 logs, each about 10 inches long, and place them on a baking sheet lined with parchment paper. Flatten each slightly to form rectangles.

4. Bake for about 20 minutes, or until firm. Let the pan cool on a rack for about 15 minutes. Turn the oven down to 300°F. Use a knife to cut each loaf diagonally into ½-inch slices. Place the slices on a baking sheet, cut sides down. Bake, turning once, until crisp, about 15 minutes. Let cool completely before serving.

Storage:
Keep in a resealable plastic bag or airtight container at room temperature for up to 5 days or freeze for up to 1 month.

Apple Pie Cookies ●

18 cookies

These cookies combine all the flavors of traditional apple pie and have a texture similar to that of a soft granola bar. A great snack!

> 1 cup old-fashioned rolled oats
> ¾ cup whole-wheat flour
> 1 teaspoon ground cinnamon
> ½ teaspoon baking powder
> Pinch of ground nutmeg
> Pinch of salt
> ¾ cup unsweetened applesauce
> ⅓ cup sugar substitute
> ⅓ cup liquid egg
> 2 teaspoons vanilla extract
> 1 apple, cored and finely diced

(continued)

1. Combine the oats, flour, cinnamon, baking powder, nutmeg, and salt in a large bowl. In another bowl, whisk together the applesauce, sugar substitute, liquid egg, and vanilla. Pour the applesauce mixture over the oat mixture and stir to combine. Add the apple and stir to distribute evenly.

2. Preheat the oven to 275°F.

3. Drop the batter by heaping tablespoonfuls onto a baking sheet lined with parchment paper. Bake until firm and lightly golden, about 25 minutes. Let cool completely.

Storage:
Keep in an airtight container for up to 3 days or freeze for up to 2 weeks.

Pecan Brownies ●

16 brownies

Brownies, you ask? That's right. These are green-light. They're packed with fiber and absolutely scrumptious, so get baking!

> *1 can (15 ounces) cannellini, kidney, or black beans,*
> *   rinsed and drained*
> *½ cup skim milk*
> *⅓ cup liquid egg*
> *¼ cup soft nonhydrogenated margarine, melted*
> *1 tablespoon vanilla extract*
> *¾ cup sugar substitute*
> *½ cup whole-wheat flour*
> *½ cup unsweetened cocoa powder*
> *1 teaspoon baking powder*
> *Pinch of salt*
> *½ cup chopped toasted pecans*

1. Put the beans in a food processor and pulse until coarsely pureed. Add the milk, liquid egg, margarine, and vanilla and puree until smooth, scraping down the sides of the bowl a few times. Set aside.

2. Preheat the oven to 350°F.

3. Combine the sugar substitute, flour, cocoa powder, baking powder, and salt in a large bowl. Pour the bean mixture over the flour mixture and stir to combine. Scrape the batter into an 8-inch square baking pan lined with parchment paper, smoothing the top. Sprinkle with the pecans.

4. Bake for about 18 minutes, or until a cake tester inserted in the center comes out clean. Let cool on a rack, then cut into squares.

Storage:
Cover with plastic wrap or store in an airtight container for up to 4 days. These can also be frozen, tightly covered, for up to 2 weeks.

Crustless Fruit-Topped Cheesecake ●

8 servings

The best part of cheesecake is the rich filling, so we've eliminated the crust and focussed on the middle and top layers. You can change the topping according to what fruit is in season.

> *16 ounces 1% cottage cheese*
> *8 ounces light cream cheese, softened*
> *1 cup nonfat, fruit-flavored yogurt with sweetener*
> *¾ cup sugar substitute*
> *¼ cup cornstarch*
> *2 egg whites*
> *1 tablespoon vanilla extract*
> *Pinch of salt*
>
> **Fruit Topping**
> *4 cups fresh raspberries, blueberries, or sliced*
>   *strawberries*
> *2 teaspoons fresh lemon juice*
> *Sugar substitute to taste*

1. Puree the cottage cheese in a food processor until very smooth. Add the cream cheese and puree until smooth and combined. Add the yogurt, sugar substitute, cornstarch, egg whites, vanilla, and salt and puree until smooth.

2. Preheat the oven to 325°F.

3. Pour the batter into a greased and parchment-lined 8- or 9-inch springform pan. Wrap the pan with aluminum foil so that the bottom and sides of the pan are covered. Place in a large roasting pan and fill the roasting pan with hot water to come halfway up the side of the springform pan.

4. Bake until the center is still slightly jiggly when the pan is tapped, about 40 minutes. Turn the oven off and run a small knife around the edge of the pan. Let the cake stand in the cooling oven for about 30 minutes more. Remove to a rack and let cool to room temperature. Cover, and refrigerate until chilled, about 2 hours.

5. *Make the Fruit Topping:* Meanwhile, in a large bowl combine the raspberries, lemon juice, and sugar substitute. Cut the cheesecake into wedges and serve with the fruit topping.

Storage:
Keep the cheesecake covered and refrigerated for up to 3 days.

Fruit and Yogurt Parfaits ●

6 servings

Homemade granola adds crunch between the creamy yogurt layers. Use whatever fruit is seasonal—blueberries, strawberries, and apples all work well. These parfaits are great for breakfast and snacks as well as for dessert.

> *2 cups old-fashioned rolled oats*
> *½ cup wheat germ*
> *⅓ cup wheat bran*
> *¼ cup slivered almonds*
> *¼ cup shelled unsalted sunflower seeds*
> *2 tablespoons sugar substitute*
> *1 tablespoon canola oil*
> *1 tablespoon water*
> *2 teaspoons grated orange zest*
> *1 teaspoon vanilla extract*
> *Pinch of salt*
> *½ cup raisins or dried cranberries*
> *32 ounces nonfat, fruit-flavored yogurt*
>   *with sweetener*
> *2 cups chopped fresh fruit or berries*

1. In a large bowl, toss together the oats, wheat germ, wheat bran, almonds, and sunflower seeds.

2. Preheat the oven to 300°F.

3. In a small bowl, whisk together the sugar substitute, oil, water, orange zest, vanilla, and salt. Pour over the oat mixture and toss well to coat evenly. Spread the mixture onto a large baking sheet lined with parchment paper and bake, stirring once, until golden brown, about 30 minutes. Let cool completely. Add the raisins, stirring to combine.

4. In a large glass serving bowl, layer 1 cup of the yogurt, then half of the granola. Repeat once and top with the remaining yogurt. Sprinkle the fruit on top.

Storage:
Cover the parfait and refrigerate for up to 2 days. Note that as the parfait sits the granola softens.

Granola Storage:
Keep in a resealable plastic bag or airtight container at room temperature for up to 3 days.

Yogurt Cheese Option:
Use Sweet Yogurt Cheese (page 279) instead of yogurt.

Almond-Crusted Pears ●

4 servings

This dessert is a great way to end a dinner party. The almonds form a crunchy crust on the outside, contrasting the tender flesh of the pears inside. Serve some of the juice from the pan alongside the pears.

1 cup plain low-fat yogurt
4 tablespoons sugar substitute
½ teaspoon grated orange zest (optional)
¾ cup sliced almonds
2 tablespoons wheat germ
4 ripe Bartlett or Bosc pears, cored and left whole
2 tablespoons liquid egg
½ cup pear nectar or juice

1. *Make the yogurt cheese:* Place the yogurt in a sieve lined with cheesecloth or with a coffee filter. Place the sieve over a bowl. Cover with plastic wrap and refrigerate for at least 1 hour or up to 4 hours. Discard the liquid that drains off and transfer the yogurt cheese to another bowl. Add 2 tablespoons of the sugar substitute and the orange zest (if using) and stir to combine. Cover with plastic wrap and refrigerate.

2. Use your hands to crush the almonds slightly, then place them in a shallow dish. Add the wheat germ and the remaining sugar substitute and stir to combine.

3. Preheat the oven to 400°F.

4. Fill the pears loosely with the almond mixture. Brush each pear with a light coating of liquid egg, then roll and press the pears into the almond mixture. Place the coated pears in an 8-inch square baking dish, standing upright. Pour the pear nectar in the bottom of the dish and sprinkle any remaining almond mixture into the pan. Cover the dish lightly with aluminum foil and bake until the pears can be pierced easily with a knife, about 30 minutes. Remove the foil and bake until the crust is golden and the juices have thickened, about 10 minutes. Let cool slightly. Serve with the yogurt cheese.

Frozen Blueberry Treat ●

3 cups

This tangy, refreshing yogurt treat tastes like a blueberry sorbet. You can make this in an ice cream machine if you have one.

> ½ cup water
> ½ cup sugar substitute
> 3 cups fresh blueberries
> 1 cup plain low-fat yogurt

1. Bring the water and sugar substitute to a boil in a saucepan over medium heat. Remove from the heat and let cool completely.

2. Meanwhile, puree the blueberries in a food processor or blender. Add the yogurt and pulse to combine. Add the sugar substitute–water mixture and pulse to combine. Pour into an 8- or 9-inch metal cake pan and freeze until firm, about 2 hours. Cut into chunks and, working in batches, place the frozen chunks in the food processor. Puree until smooth, scrape into an airtight container, and freeze until firm.

3. Before serving, place the frozen treat in the refrigerator for 15 minutes to soften slightly.

(continued)

Storage:
Keep tightly covered in the freezer for up to 1 week.

Berry Option:
Use 3 cups sliced strawberries or raspberries instead of the blueberries.

Tofu Option:
Use 1 cup of soft silken tofu instead of the yogurt.

Frozen Blueberry Option:
You can substitute 3 cups frozen blueberries for the fresh. Thaw them slightly and puree with the yogurt and water mixture. Enjoy right away or freeze—you don't have to puree the mixture again.

Fruit-Filled Pavlova ●

8 to 10 servings

Pavlovas are meringues filled with whipped cream and fruit. They are light and tasty and, thanks to the fruit, contain some fiber. The tofu and yogurt cheese we call for in place of whipped cream add protein, too.

> *8 egg whites*
> *½ teaspoon cream of tartar*
> *Pinch of salt*
> *¾ cup sugar substitute*
> *2 tablespoons cornstarch*
> *2 teaspoons vanilla extract*

Fruit Filling

1 package (14 ounces) soft silken tofu, drained
1 cup Yogurt Cheese (page 279)
¼ cup sugar substitute
½ teaspoon grated orange zest
4 cups mixed fruit (such as fresh berries and orange
*   and peach wedges)*
2 tablespoons chopped fresh mint

1. Put the egg whites in a large bowl and beat with an electric mixer until frothy. Add the cream of tartar and salt and beat until soft peaks form. Gradually add the sugar substitute and beat until the peaks become stiff. Beat in the cornstarch and vanilla to combine.

2. Preheat the oven to 275°F.

3. Spread the mixture into an 8-inch round on a baking sheet lined with parchment paper. Mound the edges slightly higher than the center to form a shell. Bake until lightly golden, about 40 minutes. Turn off the oven and let the meringue rest in the oven for 1 hour. Remove to a large serving platter.

4. *Make the Fruit Filling:* Meanwhile, in a large bowl combine the tofu, Yogurt Cheese, sugar substitute, and orange zest. Scrape into the meringue shell and top with the fruit mixture. Sprinkle with mint before serving.

Storage:
The pavlova shell can be made up to 4 hours ahead. Fill it with the fruit filling no more than 1 hour before serving.

Baked Apple ●

1 serving

I love this recipe because it's so quick and easy and you can double or triple it as need be. Baked apples make a delicious sweet snack—and they're also very healthy. You could even have this for breakfast.

> 1 apple, cored
> 3 tablespoons Muesli (page 96)
> 1 tablespoon nonhydrogenated soft margarine
> 1 tablespoon raisins
> 2 teaspoons sugar substitute
> Pinch of ground cinnamon
> Pinch of ground nutmeg

1. Place the apple on a small plate or in a bowl.

2. In a separate bowl, combine the Muesli, margarine, raisins, and sugar substitute. Stuff the mixture into the center of the apple. Press any excess filling on top of the apple. Dust with cinnamon and nutmeg. Cover loosely with plastic wrap and microwave on High until the apple is tender when pierced with a knife, about 3 minutes (see Hint).

Pear Option:
Omit the apple and use a firm, ripe Bartlett or Bosc pear. Note that the cooking time will be shorter.

Helpful Hint:
Microwave cooking times will vary depending on the wattage of your microwave. Check the apple halfway through to determine how much longer it needs to cook.

Poached Pears ●

2 servings

Poaching pears in fruit juice adds to their sweetness and gives them a richer flavor. Serve with a dollop of Yogurt Cheese (page 279) or low-fat, no-sugar-added ice cream.

> *2 cups pear juice*
> *4 black peppercorns*
> *2 whole cloves*
> *1 cinnamon stick*
> *2 pears, cored and quartered (see Hint)*

1. Bring the juice, peppercorns, cloves, and cinnamon stick to a boil in a saucepan. Reduce the heat to low and add the pears. Simmer until the pears are tender when pierced with a knife, about 10 minutes. Remove to a bowl.

2. Bring the juice mixture to a boil again. Boil for 3 minutes, then strain and drizzle over the pears.

Helpful Hint:
Look for ripe pears by picking them up and pressing gently on their skin. If a pear yields slightly and smells fresh and ripe, then that's the one you want to bring home.

Basmati Rice Pudding
with Peaches ●

4 servings

Here is quintessential comfort food to warm the heart and soul. Try serving this with other favorite fruits, such as strawberries or plums.

> *3 cups skim milk*
> *½ cup basmati rice*
> *¼ cup sugar substitute*
> *1 teaspoon vanilla extract*
> *¼ teaspoon ground cardamom or cinnamon*
> *2 peaches or nectarines, peeled, pitted, and*
>   *thinly sliced*

1. Bring the milk and rice to a boil in a heavy saucepan over medium heat. Reduce the heat to low, stir, then cover and cook until most of the milk is absorbed, about 30 minutes. Stir in the sugar substitute, vanilla, and cardamom.

2. Spoon the pudding into 4 custard cups and top with sliced peaches.

Berry Crumble ●

6 servings

This is one of my wife's favorite green-light desserts. Though it's best made with fresh berries during the summer, it's also lovely with frozen fruit.

> 5 cups fresh or frozen berries, such as raspberries,
>   blackberries, blueberries, or sliced strawberries
> 1 large apple, cored and chopped
> 2 tablespoons whole-wheat flour
> 2 tablespoons sugar substitute
> ½ teaspoon ground cinnamon
>
> **Topping**
> 1 cup old-fashioned rolled oats
> ½ cup chopped pecans or walnuts
> ¼ cup brown sugar substitute
> ¼ cup nonhydrogenated soft margarine, melted
> 1 teaspoon ground cinnamon

1. Combine the berries and apple in an 8-inch square baking dish. Combine the flour, sugar substitute, and cinnamon in a bowl. Sprinkle over the fruit and toss gently.

2. Preheat the oven to 350°F.

3. *Make the Topping:* Combine the oats, pecans, brown sugar substitute, margarine, and cinnamon in a bowl. Sprinkle over the fruit mixture. Bake until the fruit is tender and the topping is golden, about 30 minutes.

Microwave Option:
Prepare as above and microwave on High for about 6 minutes or until the fruit is tender. Be sure to use a glass, not metal, baking dish, and note that the top won't become golden or crisp in the microwave.

Glazed Apple Tart ●

6 servings

This tart deserves an audience; serve it the next time company is coming. It's especially pretty made with red-skinned apples.

1 cup whole almonds
½ cup whole-wheat cracker or dried bread crumbs
1 teaspoon ground cinnamon
2 egg whites, lightly beaten
½ cup unsweetened applesauce
1 egg
2 tablespoons sugar substitute
¼ teaspoon almond extract
2 apples, cored
2 tablespoons unsweetened apricot or peach jam

1. Preheat the oven to 350°F. Place the almonds on a baking sheet and toast until fragrant, about 10 minutes. Let cool. Keep the oven at 350°F.

2. Put the almonds in a food processor and pulse until they are ground fine. Transfer them to a bowl. Add the cracker crumbs and ½ teaspoon of the cinnamon and toss to combine. Add the egg whites and stir to combine. Press the mixture into the bottom and up the sides of an 8-inch pie plate. Bake for about 10 minutes, or until firm. Let cool. Turn the oven up to 400°F.

3. In a bowl, whisk together the applesauce, egg, sugar substitute, remaining cinnamon, and almond extract. Spread this over the crust.

4. Cut each apple in half and cut each half into thin half-moon-shaped slices. Place the slices in concentric circles over the applesauce mixture. Bake for about 15 minutes, or until the apples are tender when pierced with knife. Brush the apple slices with jam. Let cool on a rack.

Baked Chocolate Mousse ●

4 servings

This mousse is so dense and rich it seems sinful. But no worries, it's green-light. Make it on the weekend to enjoy throughout the week.

1 cup skim milk
3 ounces unsweetened chocolate, chopped
½ cup liquid egg
1 cup sugar substitute
2 teaspoons vanilla extract

1. Heat the milk in a saucepan over medium heat until steaming. Whisk in the chocolate and cook until melted.

2. Preheat the oven to 325°F.

3. In a bowl, whisk together the liquid egg, sugar substitute, and vanilla. Gradually whisk the milk mixture into the egg mixture until combined. Pour into 4 custard cups or ramekins and place the cups in a baking dish. Fill the baking dish with enough boiling water to come halfway up the sides of the custard cups.

4. Bake for about 25 minutes, or until a knife inserted in the center of a mousse comes out creamy.

Storage:
Let cool completely before refrigerating so no water droplets form on the surface of the mousse. Cover with plastic wrap and refrigerate for up to 1 week.

Part Four

Appendices

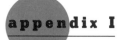

The Green-Light Glossary

The following is a summary of the most popular green-light foods.

Almonds This is the perfect nut in that it has the highest monounsaturated fat (good fat) content of any nut, and recent research indicates that almonds can significantly lower LDL (bad) cholesterol. They are also excellent sources of vitamin E, fiber, and protein. They provide a great boost to the beneficial fat content of your meals, especially at breakfast or in salads and desserts. Because all nuts are high in calories, use them in moderation.

Apples A real staple. Use fresh for a snack or dessert. Unsweetened applesauce is ideal with cereals or with cottage cheese.

Barley An easy-to-cook grain filled with fiber and nutrients. An excellent supplement to soups.

Beans (legumes) If there's one food you can never get enough of, it's beans. These perfect green-light foods are high in protein and fiber and can supplement nearly every meal.

Make bean salads or just add beans to any salad. Add to soups, replace some of the meat in casseroles, or add to meat loaf. Serve them as a side vegetable or as an alternative to potatoes, rice, or pasta. Check out the wide range of canned and frozen beans.

Exercise caution with baked beans, as the sauce can be high-fat and high-calorie. Ditto for refried beans. Check labels for low-fat versions and watch your serving size.

Beans have a well-deserved reputation for creating "wind," so be patient until your body adapts—as it will—to your increased consumption.

Bread Most breads are red-light except for coarse or stone-ground, 100% whole-wheat, or whole-grain breads. Check labels carefully, as the bread industry likes to confuse the unwary. "Stone-ground 100% whole wheat" is the wording to look for. With other breads, look for at least 3 grams of fiber per slice.

Most bread is made from flour ground by steel rollers that strip away the bran coating. Stone-ground flour retains more of its bran coating, so it is digested more slowly in your stomach.

Even with stone-ground, 100% whole-wheat bread, watch your quantity—one slice per serving. Use sparingly where you cannot avoid it, such as lunch in Phase I, and only occasionally in Phase II.

Cereals Use only large-flake oats, oat bran, or high-fiber cold cereals (10 grams of fiber per serving or higher). Though these cereals are not much fun in themselves, you can dress them up with fruit (fresh, frozen, or canned) or with fruit-flavored fat-free yogurt with sweetener. This way, you can change the menu daily. Use sweetener, not sugar.

Cottage cheese Fat-free or 1% cottage cheese is an excellent low-fat, high-protein food. Add fruit to make a snack or add it to salads.

Eggs By far the best options are egg whites or eggs in liquid form (packaged in a carton), which are virtually cholesterol- and fat-free. In Phase II, if you'd really rather use whole eggs, buy the omega-3 kind, which are beneficial for heart health.

Fish/shellfish These are ideal green-light foods, low in fat and cholesterol and a good source of protein. Some coldwater fish such as salmon are rich in omega-3 oils. Never eat battered or breaded fish.

Food bars Most food or nutrition bars are a dietary disaster, high in carbohydrates and calories but low in protein. These bars are quick sugar fixes on the run. There are a few, such as Balance, that have a more equitable distribution of carbohydrates, proteins, and fats. Look for 20 to 30 grams of carbohydrates, 12 to 15 grams of protein, and 4 to 6 grams of fat. This equals about 220 calories per bar.

    Serving size for a snack is one half of a bar. Keep one in your office desk or your purse for a convenient on-the-run snack. In an emergency, I have been known to have one bar plus an apple and a glass of skim milk for lunch when a proper lunch break was impossible. This is okay in emergencies, but don't make a habit of it.

Grapefruit One of the top-rated green-light foods. Eat as often as you like.

Hamburgers These are acceptable but only with extra-lean ground beef that has 10 percent or less fat. Mix in some oat bran to reduce the meat content but keep the bulk.

A better option would be to replace the beef with ground turkey or chicken breast. And there are some soy substitutes for meat that are low in fat—they taste remarkably good and are worth checking out. Keep the serving size at 4 ounces; use only half of a whole-wheat bun and eat open-faced.

Ice cream Look for low-fat, no-sugar-added varieties, with 90 to 100 calories per ½-cup serving. And stick to this maximum serving size despite the temptation!

Meat The best green-light meats are skinless chicken and turkey, fully trimmed beef, veal, deli cuts of lean ham, and Canadian bacon. The beef cuts to choose are eye of round and top round. For pork, choose tenderloin.

Milk Use skim only. If you have trouble adjusting, then use 1% and slowly wean yourself off it. The fat you're giving up is saturated (bad) fat. Milk is a terrific snack or meal supplement. I drink two glasses of skim milk a day, at breakfast and lunch.

Nuts A principal source of "good" fat, which is essential for your health. Almonds are your best choice, but cashews, hazelnuts, macadamia nuts, and pistachios are also green-light. Add them to cereals, salads, and desserts. As they are calorie-dense, use in moderation.

Oat bran An excellent high-fiber additive to baking as a partial replacement for flour. Also great as a hot cereal.

Oatmeal If you haven't had oatmeal since you were a kid, now's the time to revisit it. Large-flake or old-fashioned oatmeal is the breakfast of choice, with the added advantage for your heart of lowering cholesterol. The instant and quick-cooking (one-minute) versions are not recommended—they have a higher G.I. rating due to the extra processing of the oats. A somewhat cynical colleague recently decided to take my advice about the G.I. Diet, but only a meal at a time, starting with oatmeal for breakfast. His oatmeal-based green-light breakfast has so far netted him 10 pounds of weight loss! He's since thrown caution to the wind and is now a convert to three green-light meals a day. Personally, I often have hot oatmeal with unsweetened applesauce and sweetener as a snack on weekends (I use ⅓ cup dry oats).

Oranges Whole or in segments, fresh oranges are excellent as snacks, on cereal, and especially at breakfast. A glass of orange juice has two and a half times as many calories as a whole orange, so avoid the juice and stick with the real thing.

Pasta There are two golden rules. First, do not overcook; al dente (some firmness to the bite) is important. Second, serving size is key; pasta is a side dish and should never occupy more than a quarter of your plate. It *must not* form the basis of the meal, as it most commonly does nowadays in America, with disastrous results for waistlines and hips. Whole-wheat pasta is preferable.

Peaches/pears/plums Terrific snacks, desserts, or additions to breakfast cereal. Use them fresh, or canned in juice or water (not syrup).

Potatoes The only form of potatoes that is acceptable even on an occasional basis is boiled new potatoes. New potatoes have a low starch content, unlike larger, more mature potatoes that have been allowed to build their starch levels. All other forms of potato—baked, mashed, or fried—are strictly red-light. Limit the quantity to two or three new potatoes per serving.

Rice There is a wide range in the G.I. ratings for various types of rice, most of which are red-light. The best rice is basmati or long-grain, which is readily available at your supermarket. Brown rice is better than white. If rice is sticky, with the grains clumping together, don't use it. Similarly, don't overcook rice; the more it's cooked, the more glutinous and therefore unacceptable it becomes. The rule, then, is eat only slightly undercooked basmati or long-grain rice.

Root vegetables Most root vegetables, such as yams, sweet potatoes, beets, parsnips, and rutabaga, are red- or yellow-light, principally because of their high G.I. and starch content. Accordingly, yellow-light root vegetables should be used in moderation in Phase II. However, carrots, with their low carbohydrate content, are green-light.

Soups I recommend that all soups be made from scratch, as commercial soups are subjected to high temperatures in the canning process to kill bacteria, which raises the G.I. If convenience is important, then the brands listed on page 22 are the best choices among the commercial soups.

Sour cream One percent or nonfat sour cream with a little sweetener stirred in is an ideal alternative to whipped cream as a dessert topping. You can also mix fruit or low-sugar fruit spread into it for a creamy dessert.

Soy Soy protein powder is a simple way to boost the protein level of any meal. It's particularly useful at breakfast for sprinkling over cereal. Look for the kind that has a 90 percent protein content. It's sometimes labeled "isolated soy protein powder." Unflavored low- or nonfat soy milk is a perfect green-light beverage.

Sushi Fish is an excellent green-light food. However, the rice normally served with sushi is glutinous and high-G.I. So eat the fish, but minimize the rice—stick with the sashimi options on the menu. If preparing at home, use basmati or long-grain rice. Prepared sushi rolls with their high rice content are not a good idea.

Sweeteners There has been a tremendous amount of misinformation circulating about artificial sweeteners—all of which has proven groundless. The sugar industry rightly sees these products as a threat and has done its best to bad-mouth them. You can find an excellent medical overview of sugar substitutes at the U.S. Food and Drug Administration's Web site (www.fda.gov). Use sweeteners to replace sugar wherever possible. Splenda is our preferred choice. If you are allergic to sweeteners, then fructose is a better alternative to sucrose (cane sugar). Use the herbal sweetener stevia (found in health food stores) in moderation, as no long-term studies on its use are available.

Tofu Though not flavorful in itself, tofu is an excellent low-fat source of protein. Use it to boost or replace meat or seafood in dishes such as salads, burgers, and stir-fries.

Yogurt Fat-free fruit-flavored yogurt with sweetener is a near-perfect green-light product. It's an ideal snack food on its own, or a flavorful addition to breakfast cereal—especially hot oatmeal—and to fruit for dessert. Our fridge is always full of it, in half a dozen delicious flavors. In fact, my shopping cart is usually so full of yogurt containers that fellow shoppers frequently stop me to ask if they are on special!

Yogurt Cheese Easy to prepare (see page 279), it's a wonderful substitute for cream in desserts or in main dishes like chili (see pages 176 and 226).

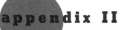

Green-Light Kitchen Cupboard Essentials

PANTRY

baking/cooking

Baking powder/soda
Cocoa (70%)
Dried apricots
Sliced almonds
Wheat/oat bran
Whole-wheat flour

beans (canned)

Baked beans (low-fat)
Mixed salad beans
Soybeans
Vegetarian chili

breads

100% stone-ground
whole-wheat

cereals

All-Bran
Bran Buds
Fiber One
Kashi Go Lean
Oatmeal (large-flake)

drinks

Bottled water
Club soda
Decaffeinated
coffee/tea
Diet decaffeinated
soft drinks

fats/oils

Canola oil
Margarine
(soft, light)
Mayonnaise
(nonfat)
Olive oil
Salad dressings
Vegetable oil spray

fruit (canned/bottled)

Applesauce
(unsweetened)
Mandarin oranges
Peaches in juice or water
Pears in juice or water

pasta (whole-wheat)

Fettuccine
Spaghetti
Vermicelli

pasta sauces (vegetable-based only)

Healthy Choice

rice

Basmati, long-grain,
wild

seasonings

Flavored vinegars/
sauces
Spices/herbs

snacks

Food bars (Balance)

soups (vegetable- or bean-based only)

Healthy Choice
Healthy Request

sweeteners

Equal
Splenda
Sugar Twin
Sweet'n Low

vegetables

Potatoes
(new, small only)
Tomatoes

FRIDGE

dairy

Buttermilk
Cottage cheese (1%)
Fruit yogurt (nonfat
with sweetener)
Milk (skim)
Sour cream
(nonfat or 1%)

fruit

Apples
Blackberries
Blueberries
Cherries
Grapefruit
Grapes
Lemons
Limes
Oranges
Peaches
Pears
Plums
Raspberries
Strawberries

meat/poultry/ fish/eggs

Chicken breast
(skinless)
Ground beef
(extra-lean)
Ham/turkey/chicken
(lean deli)
Liquid eggs/egg whites
Seafood, fresh, frozen,
or canned in water
(no batter or breading)
Turkey breast
(skinless)
Veal

vegetables

Asparagus
Beans (green or wax)
Bell peppers
Broccoli

Cabbage
Carrots
Cauliflower
Celery
Cucumber
Eggplant
Leeks
Lettuce
Mushrooms
Olives
Onions
Peppers (hot)
Pickles
Radishes
Snow peas
Spinach
Tomatoes
Zucchini

FREEZER

dairy

Frozen yogurt (nonfat
and no sugar added)
Ice cream (nonfat and
no sugar added)

snacks

Homemade muffins
(see pages 261 to 268)

vegetables/fruit

Mixed berries
Mixed peppers
Mixed vegetables
Peas

G.I. Diet Shopping List

PANTRY

baking/cooking

- [ ] Baking powder/soda
- [ ] Cocoa (70%)
- [ ] Dried apricots
- [ ] Sliced almonds
- [ ] Wheat/oat bran
- [ ] Whole-wheat flour

beans (canned)

- [ ] Baked beans (low-fat)
- [ ] Most varieties
- [ ] Mixed salad beans
- [ ] Vegetarian chili

bread

- [ ] 100% stone-ground whole-wheat

cereals

- [ ] All-Bran
- [ ] Bran Buds
- [ ] Fiber One
- [ ] Kashi Go Lean
- [ ] Oatmeal (large-flake)
- [ ] Soy protein powder

drinks

- [ ] Bottled water
- [ ] Club soda
- [ ] Decaffeinated coffee/tea
- [ ] Diet decaffeinated soft drinks

fats/oils

- [ ] Canola oil
- [ ] Margarine (soft, light)
- [ ] Mayonnaise (nonfat)
- [ ] Olive oil
- [ ] Salad dressings
- [ ] Vegetable oil spray

fruit (canned/bottled)

- [ ] Applesauce (unsweetened)
- [ ] Mandarin oranges
- [ ] Peaches in juice or water
- [ ] Pears in juice or water

pasta (whole-wheat)

- [ ] Capellini
- [ ] Fettuccine
- [ ] Macaroni
- [ ] Penne
- [ ] Spaghetti
- [ ] Vermicelli

pasta sauces (vegetable-based only)

☐ Healthy Choice

rice

☐ Basmati
☐ Long-grain
☐ Wild

seasonings

☐ Flavored vinegars/sauces

_____
_____
_____
_____
_____

☐ Spices/herbs

_____
_____
_____
_____
_____

snacks

☐ Food bars (Balance)

soups

☐ Healthy Choice
☐ Healthy Request

sweeteners

☐ Equal, Splenda, Sugar Twin, Sweet'n Low (or other non-sugar sweetener)

FRIDGE/ FREEZER

dairy

☐ Buttermilk
☐ Cottage cheese (1%)
☐ Frozen yogurt (nonfat and no sugar added)
☐ Fruit yogurt (fat-free with sweetener)
☐ Ice cream (low-fat and no sugar added)
☐ Milk (skim)
☐ Sour cream (fat-free or 1%)

fruit

☐ Apples
☐ Blackberries
☐ Blueberries
☐ Cherries
☐ Grapefruit
☐ Grapes
☐ Lemons
☐ Limes
☐ Oranges
☐ Peaches
☐ Pears
☐ Plums
☐ Raspberries
☐ Strawberries

meat/poultry/ fish/eggs

☐ Chicken breast (skinless)

☐ Ground beef (extra-lean)
☐ Ham/turkey/chicken (lean deli)
☐ Liquid eggs/ egg whites
☐ Seafood, fresh, frozen, or canned in water (no batter or breading)
☐ Turkey breast (skinless)
☐ Veal

vegetables

☐ Asparagus
☐ Beans (green/wax)
☐ Bell and hot peppers
☐ Broccoli
☐ Cabbage
☐ Carrots
☐ Cauliflower
☐ Celery
☐ Cucumber
☐ Eggplant
☐ Leeks
☐ Lettuce
☐ Mushrooms
☐ Olives
☐ Onions
☐ Pickles
☐ Potatoes (new, small only)
☐ Snow peas
☐ Spinach
☐ Tomatoes
☐ Zucchini

Dining Out and Travel Tips

	● RED LIGHT	● GREEN LIGHT
breakfast	Bacon/sausage Bagels Cold cereals Eggs Muffins Pancakes/waffles	All-Bran Egg whites/Egg Beaters—Omelet (no cheese, please) Egg whites/Egg Beaters—Scrambled Fruit Oatmeal Yogurt—nonfat with sweetener
lunch	Bakery products Butter/mayonnaise Cheese Fast food Pasta-based meals Pizza/bread/bagels Potatoes (replace with double vegetables)	Meats—deli ham, chicken, or turkey breast Pasta—¼ plate maximum Salads—low-fat (dressing on the side) Sandwiches—open-face, whole-wheat Soups—chunky vegetable and bean Vegetables Wraps—½ pita or low-carb tortilla, no mayonnaise

	● RED LIGHT	● GREEN LIGHT
dinner	Beef/lamb/pork Bread Butter/mayonnaise Caesar salad Desserts—pastries, ice cream, candy Pasta-based meals Potatoes (replace with vegetables) Soups—cream-based White rice (regular)	Chicken/turkey (no skin) Fruit Pasta—¼ plate Rice (basmati, brown, long-grain, wild)—¼ plate Salads—low-fat (dressing on the side) Seafood—not breaded or battered Soups—chunky vegetable or bean Vegetables
snacks	Candy Chips (all types) Cookies/muffins Popcorn (regular) Pretzels	Almonds Fresh fruit Hazelnuts Light cottage cheese with unsweetened fruit preserves Yogurt—nonfat with sweetener ½ food bar (e.g., Balance)

PORTIONS

Meat/fish	Palm of hand/deck of cards
Vegetables	Minimum ½ plate
Rice/pasta	Maximum ¼ plate
New potatoes	2 to 3 in Phase I; 3 to 4 in Phase II

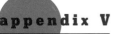

The Ten Golden G.I. Diet Rules

1. Eat three meals and three snacks every day. Don't skip meals—particularly breakfast.

2. In Phase I, stick with green-light products only.

3. When it comes to food, quantity is as important as quality. Shrink your usual portions, particularly of meat, pasta, and rice.

4. Always ensure that each meal contains the appropriate measure of carbohydrates, protein, and fat.

5. Eat at least three times more vegetables and fruit than usual.

6. Drink plenty of fluids, preferably water.

7. Exercise for thirty minutes once a day or fifteen minutes twice a day. Get off the bus or subway two stops early or park your car a mile from your destination.

8. Find a friend to join you for mutual support.

9. Set realistic goals. Try to lose an average of a pound a week and record your progress to reinforce your sense of achievement.

10. Don't view this as a diet. It's the basis of how you will eat for the rest of your life.

G.I. DIET WEEKLY WEIGHT/WAIST LOG

week	date	weight	waist	comments
1.				
2.				
3.				
4.				
5.				
6.				
7.				
8.				
9.				
10.				
11.				
12.				
13.				
14.				
15.				
16.				
17.				
18.				
19.				
20.				

G.I. DIET WEEKLY WEIGHT/WAIST LOG

week	date	weight	waist	comments
21.				
22.				
23.				
24.				
25.				
26.				
27.				
28.				
29.				
30.				
31.				
32.				
33.				
34.				
35.				
36.				
37.				
38.				
39.				
40.				

G.I. DIET WEEKLY WEIGHT/WAIST LOG

week	date	weight	waist	comments
1.				
2.				
3.				
4.				
5.				
6.				
7.				
8.				
9.				
10.				
11.				
12.				
13.				
14.				
15.				
16.				
17.				
18.				
19.				
20.				

G.I. DIET WEEKLY WEIGHT/WAIST LOG

week	date	weight	waist	comments
21.				
22.				
23.				
24.				
25.				
26.				
27.				
28.				
29.				
30.				
31.				
32.				
33.				
34.				
35.				
36.				
37.				
38.				
39.				
40.				

Notes

Notes

Index